the Same sex Kama Sutra

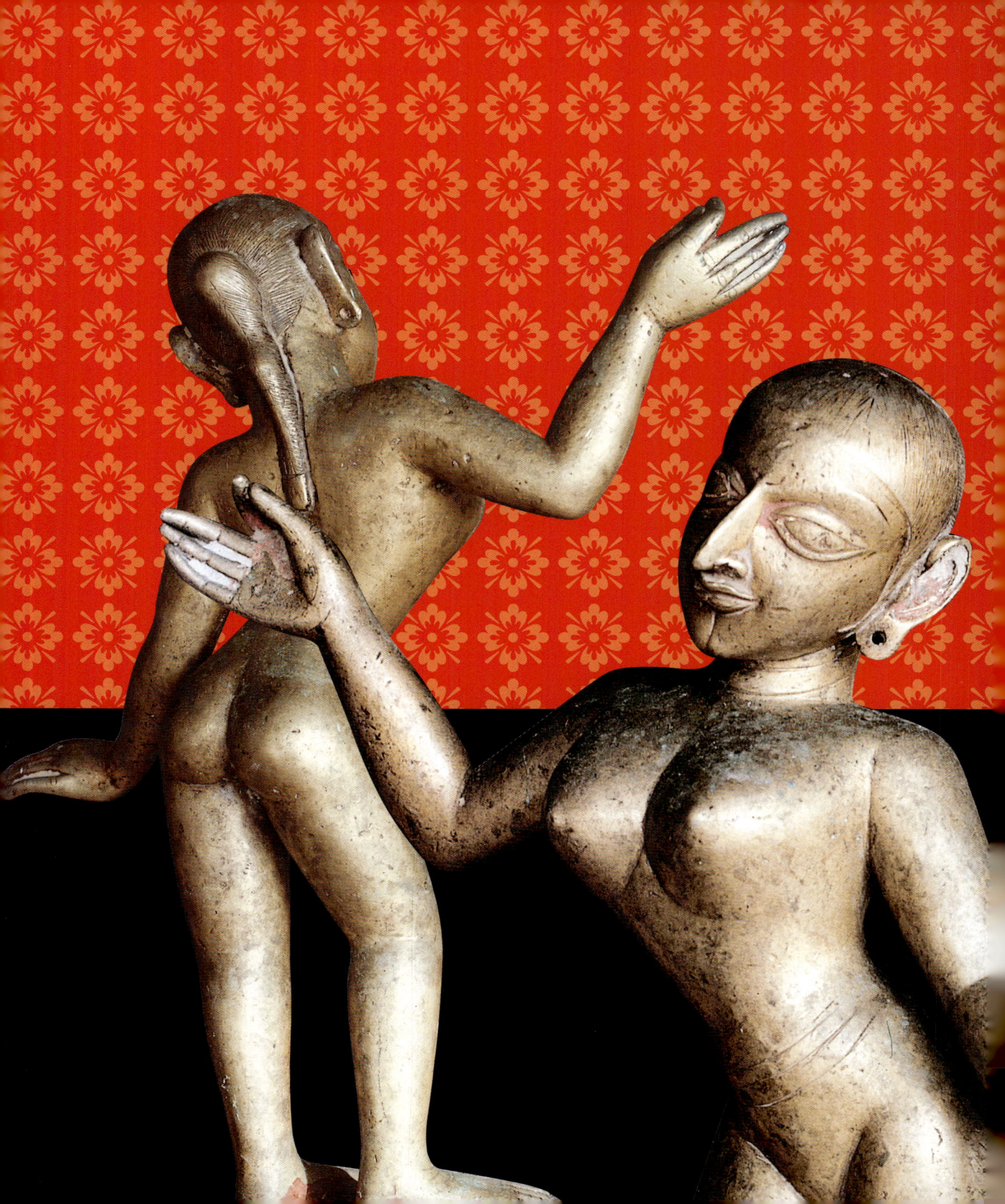

the **S**ame sex
Kama**S**utra

SANDHYA MULCHANDANI

Lustre Press
Roli Books

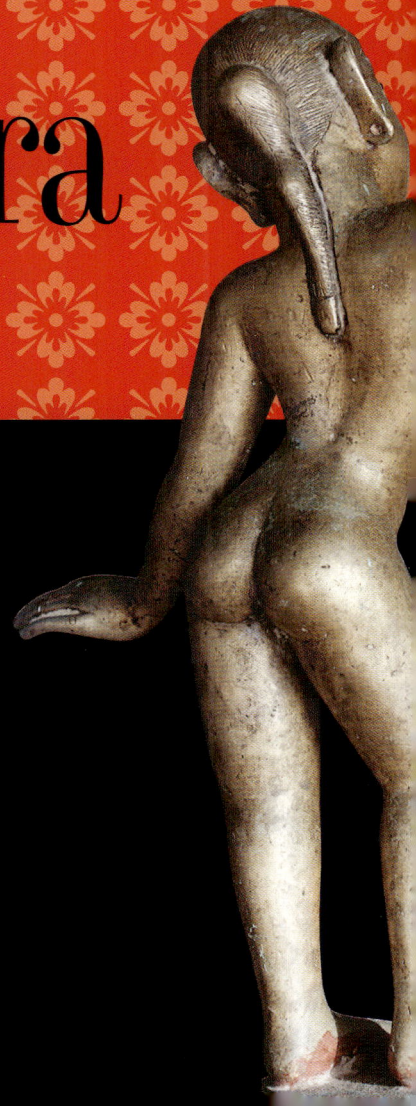

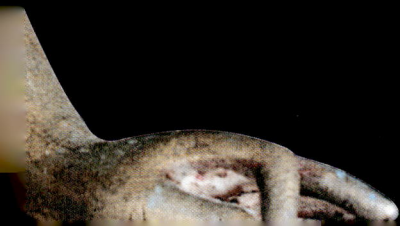

ISBN: 81-7436-385-8

© **Roli & Janssen BV 2006**
Published in India by Roli Books in arrangement with
Roli & Janssen BV, The Netherlands
M-75, Greater Kailash-II Market, New Delhi 110 048, India.
Phone: ++91-11-29212271, 29212782, Fax: ++91-11-29217185
Email: roli@vsnl.com Website: rolibooks.com

Printed and bound in Singapore

Photo credits:

Corbis: 26,-27, 66, 69, 73, 78
D.N. Dube: 88
Fitzwilliam Museum, University Of Cambridge: 81
Lance Dane: 2, 3, 5, 8, 9, 23, 36-37, 84, 114, 121, 124-125
Private Collection: 122
Roli Books Private Collection: 13, 16-17, 20, 28, 34-35, 40-41,
46-49, 54, 59-61, 65, 82, 83, 87, 91, 102, 105
Sandhya Mulchandani: 45, 92-95, Back cover
Usha Kris: 38
Victoria & Albert Museum, London: 42, 53, 77
Werner Forman Archive: 6-7, 10. 116-117

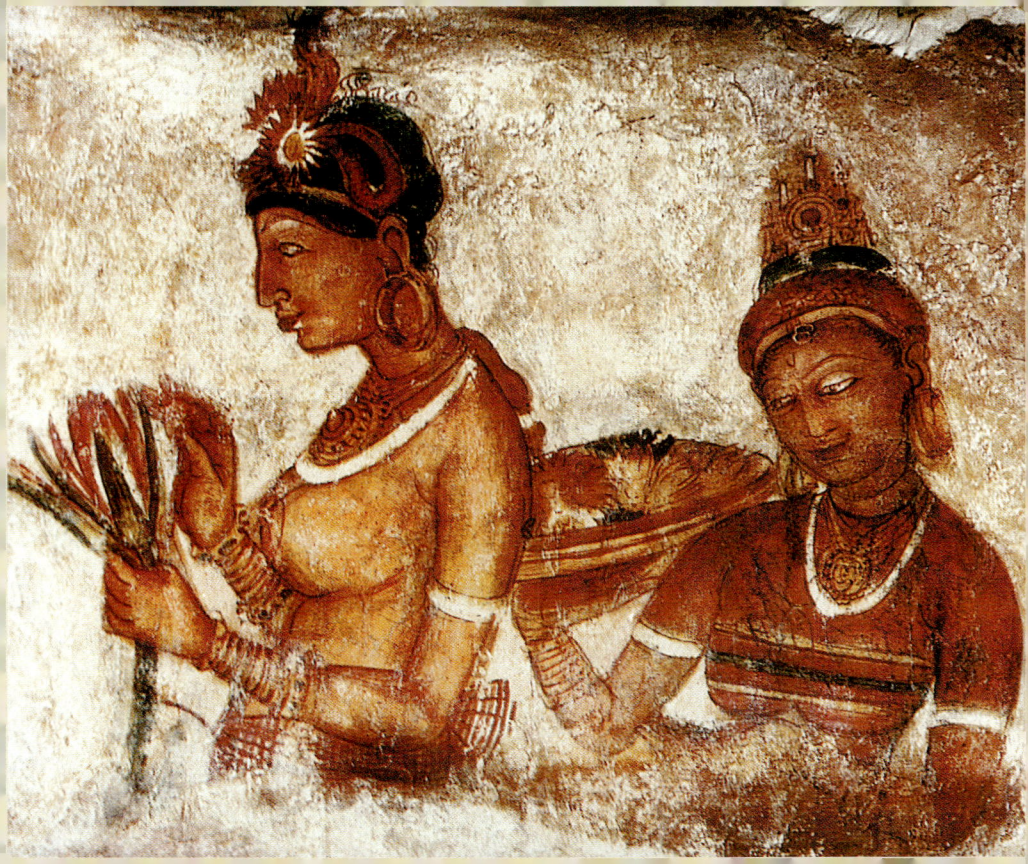

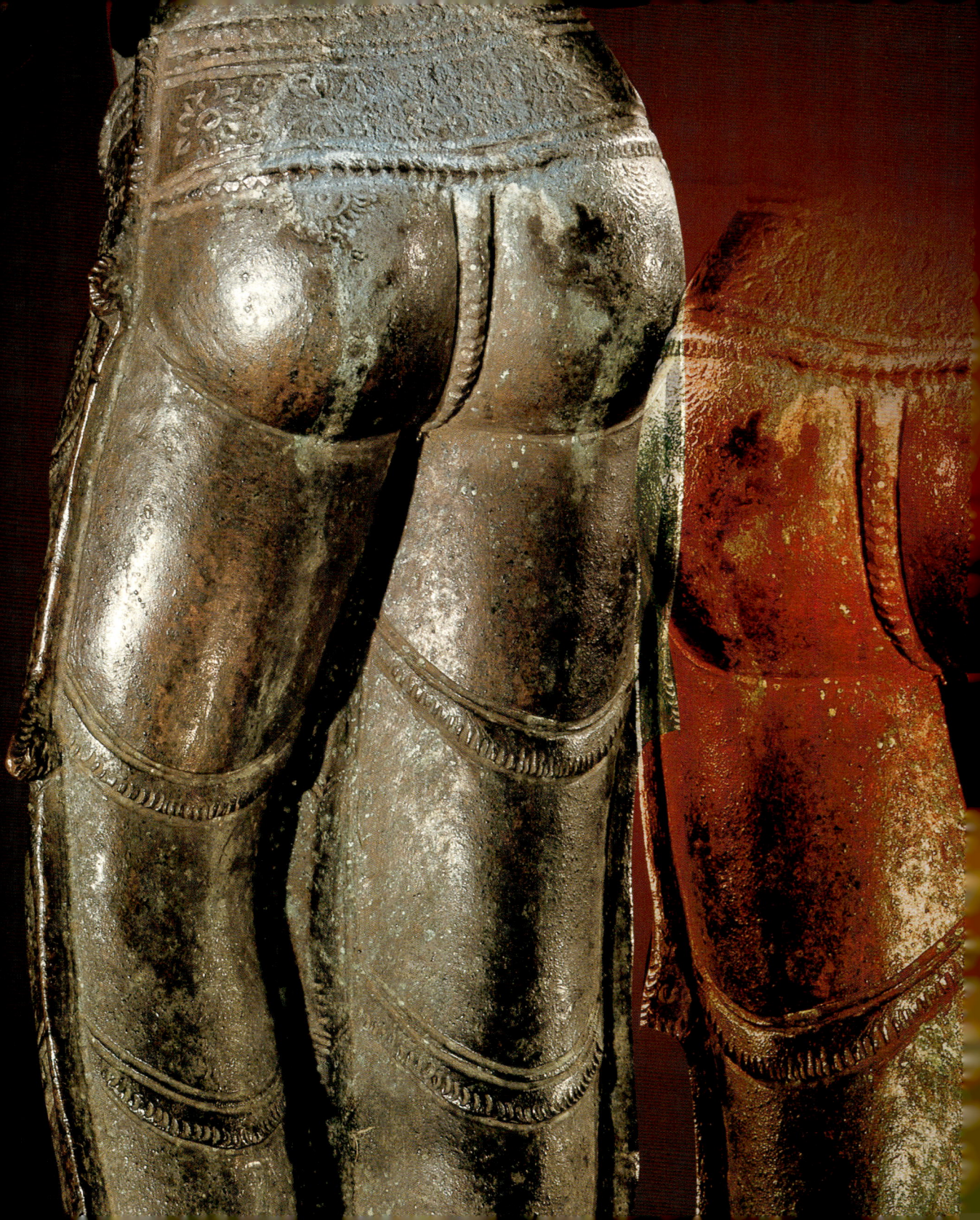

Contents

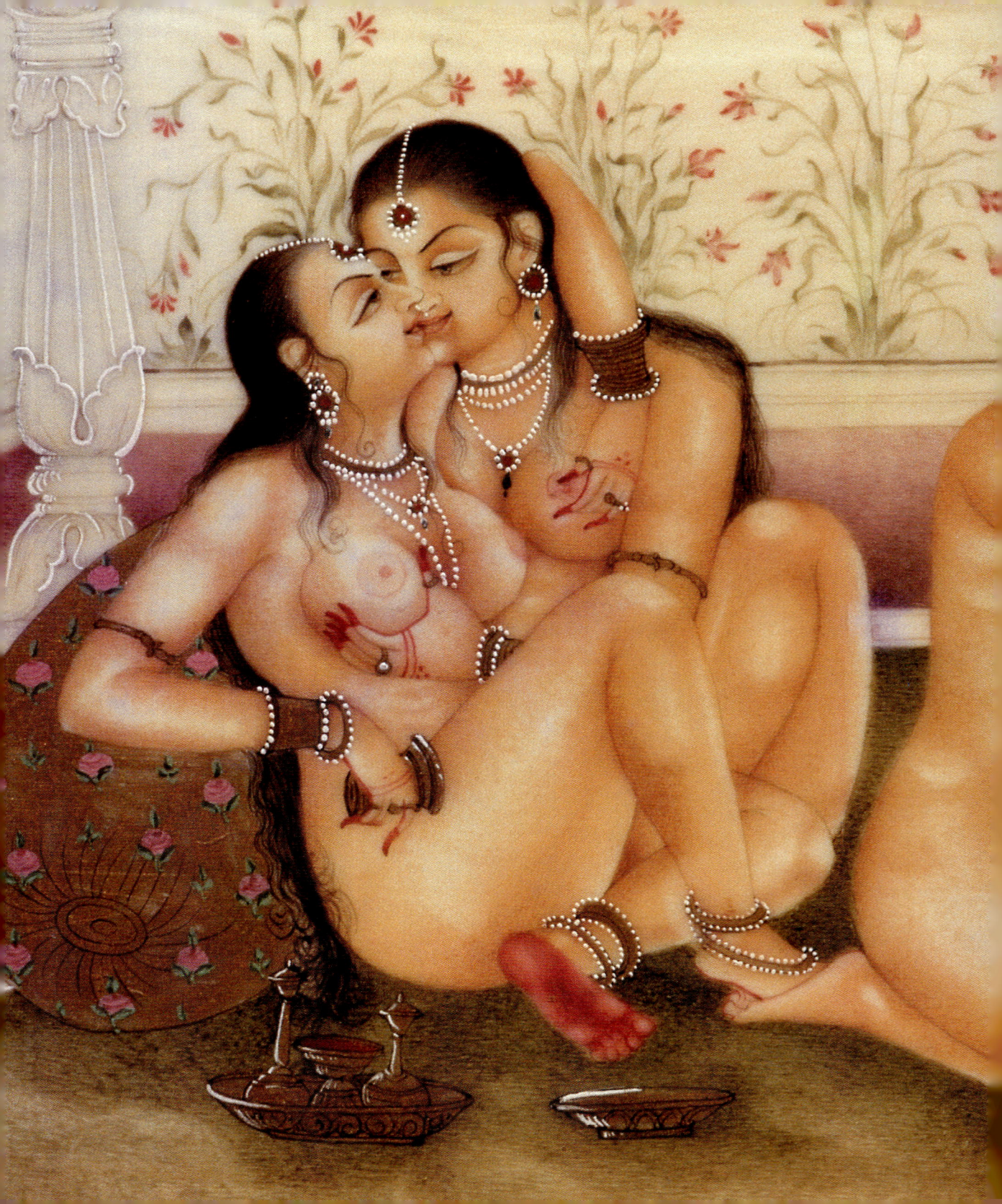

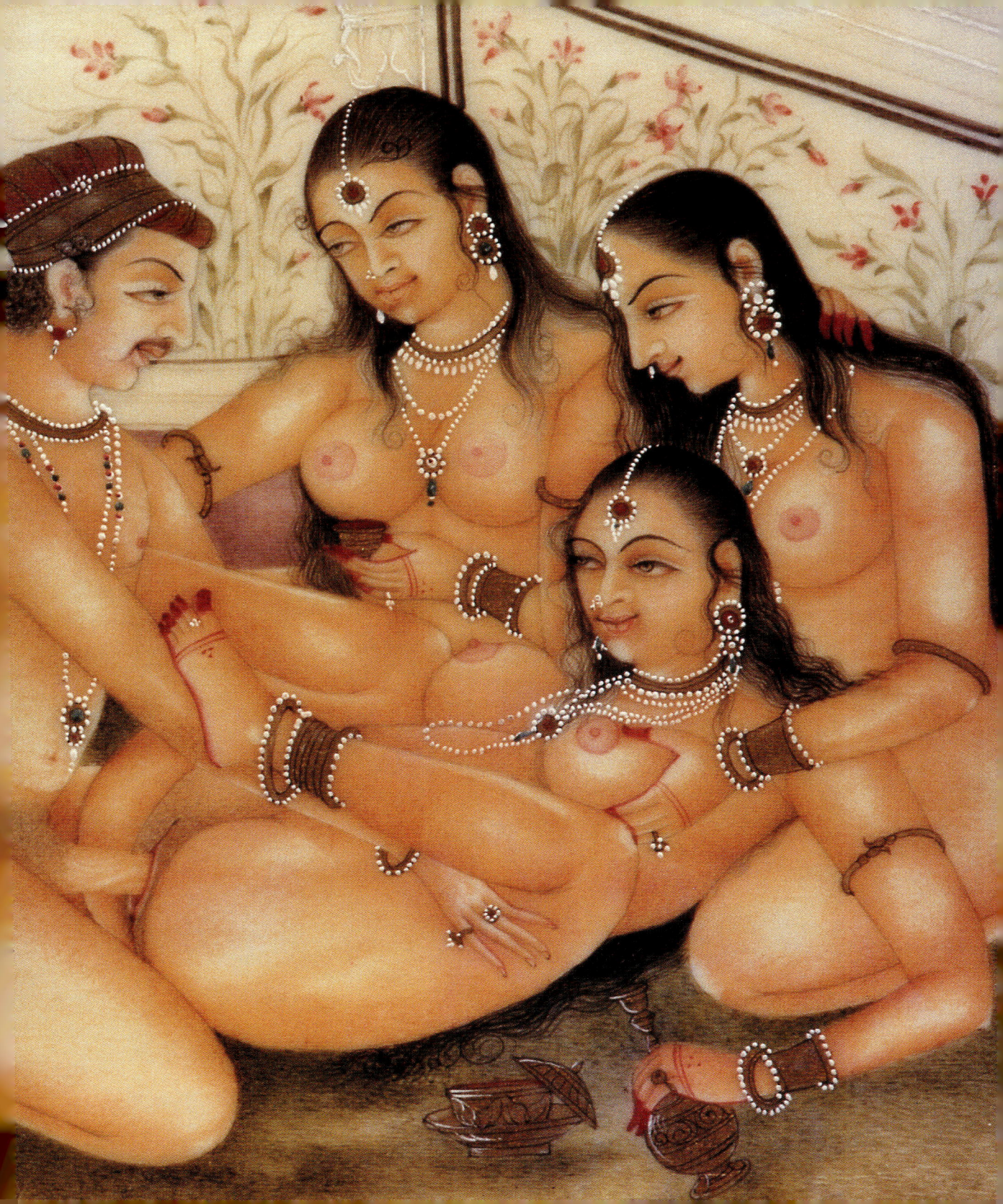

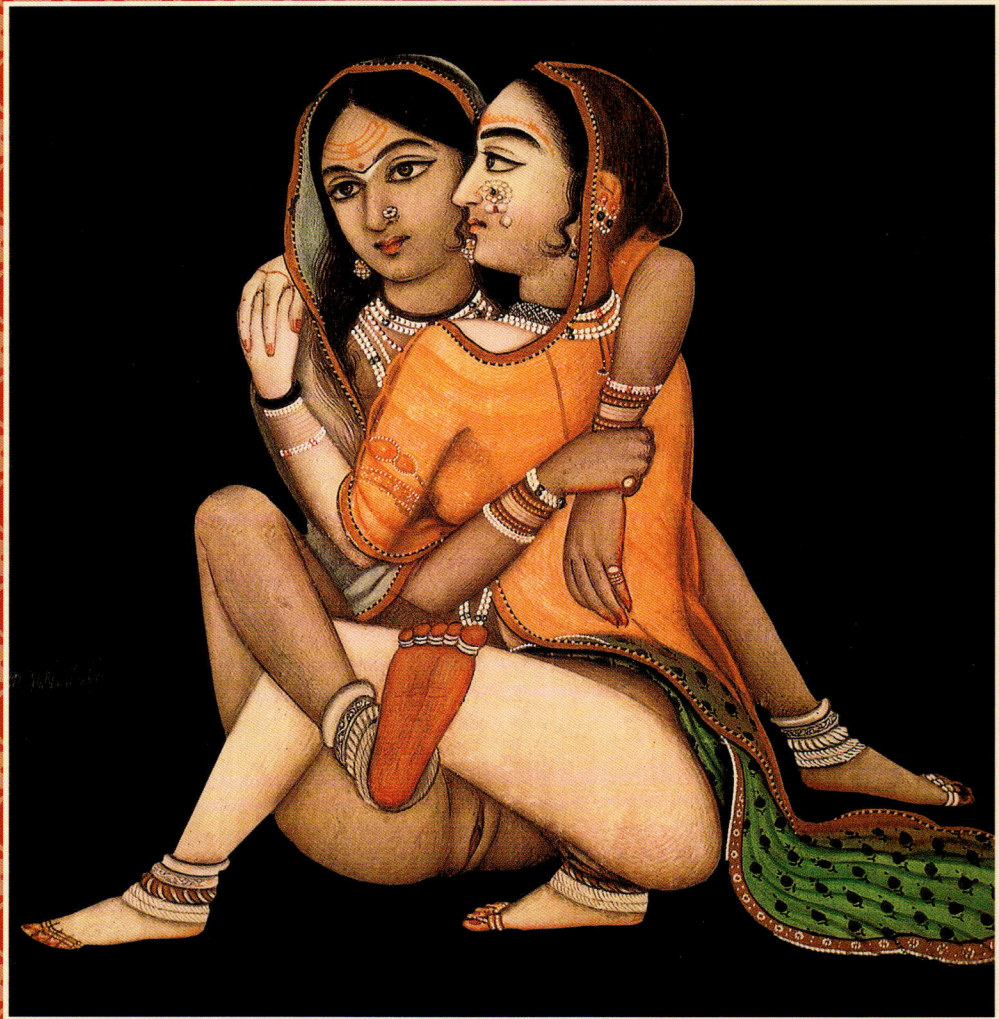

Introduction

Science and religion represent two of the world's greatest systems of thought that have stood resolutely opposed to one another. Now it would appear the two are finally headed, if not towards reconciliation, then at least towards concurrence. Increasingly Quantum physicists are affirming Eastern theology's belief that the universe was essentially created out of nothing. This emptiness, the sages believed was latent Consciousness that became manifest as the process of creation from which emerged the miracle of human awareness. This process of creation is brilliantly illustrated in several ancient mythologies but the most definitive account appears in the *Nasadiya Suktam* in the 129th hymn in the 10th chapter of the *Rg Veda*.

The Vedas, ancient Indian texts, complied around 1500 BC describe creation as an eternally magnificent, dynamic, efficient and perfect awareness that has the potential to manifest itself, repeatedly, in infinitely diverse ways. Thus the universe that emerged from this singularity—the pantheon of gods, the swirling clouds of gas, the planets and stars, the trees, flowers and blades of grass, the cuckoo and the camel, land and water, woman and man—are all mere representations of the multiplicity that we call life. The ability to accept diversity, to see it as an emanation from a single Consciousness, as well as the quest to become one with the divine life force, forms the bedrock of Hindu thought:

See unity in diversity. Behold the one divine form appearing in the multiform; Immense is His vastness, unparalleled is His glory. All the countless earths, suns and planets which are seen, and which are beyond our perception, exist under His command. Kindled in various forms, the perennial flame is one; sprinkling the world with golden beams at dawn; painting the evening clouds with changing colours, the sun is one.

(*Rg Veda* 8.58.2)

The accepted philosophy is that the universe beats to one cadence and dances to one divine tune, but diversity appears to have been mandated from first creation. Given the fluidity of the cosmos, the universe was never meant to be homogenous, making the rather utopian ideal of a world in which there is uniformity of race and colour, cast and creed, go against the grain of the principle of creation. This is particularly true in Hindu philosophy that takes pride both in its expansiveness and inclusiveness. Unity here does not stand for sameness or even uniformity; the unity that the ancient Hindus believed in was not one that forcibly brought together disparate elements which in the process obliterated different beliefs and traditions; rather it was the ability to be all encompassing—to accept and tolerate everything and view it as God's creation. The facility to understand that there is only one

---

Facing page: Divergent sexual proclivities were always a part of human nature.

ultimate Reality however divergent the *margas* or paths one chooses to follow, is an intrinsic part of what being a Hindu means.

Given the extent of diversity that exists in nature, ancient civilizations sought to relate themselves to the wonder of the universe and learnt not only to appreciate a world filled with multiplicity but also to venerate it. The story of genesis according to Hindu mythology is that the First-Born called Prajapathi felt afraid and split into two, creating woman out of his own body. Amazed at the beautiful woman standing in front of him, he lusted after her, and from this coupling followed the rest of creation making the universe not just sacred but essentially sexual as well. So, any spiritual text or theology that purported to enlighten or explain the whole of the human race had necessarily to deal with the sexual dimensions of human lives.

Hinduism though known for its extremely liberal attitude and inclusiveness, functioned within the accepted heterosexual environment. Most of its scriptures, and texts like the *Manusmriti, Dharma Shastra,* the *Griha Shastras,* focus on heterosexual relationships with monogamy, marriage and procreation being the *raison d'être* of most relationships. Ancient societies that saw the universe as an inseparable web whose interconnections were dynamic ever growing and changing, were reluctant to draw rigid moral lines, especially when they recognized that sexuality was not something that existed in convenient watertight compartments.

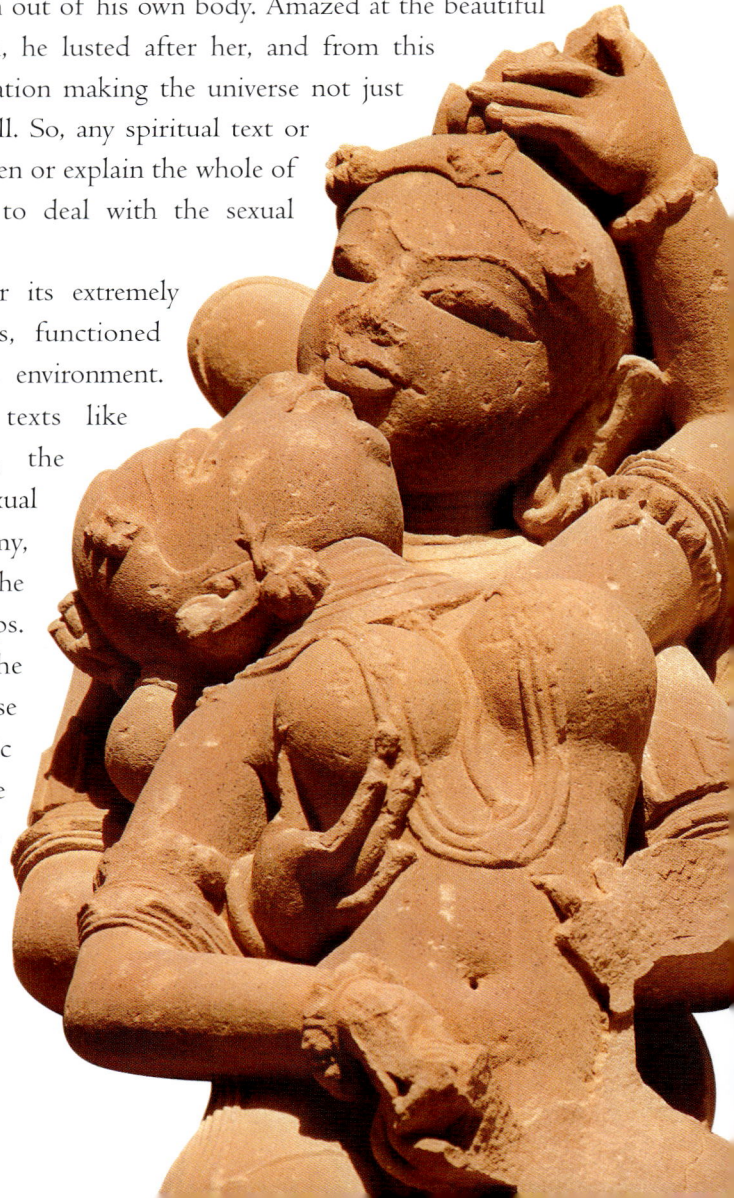

Nature has ensured a certain amount of sexual ambiguity in all living beings. It is this diversity that forms the basis of human individuation and gives man the liberty to explore and seek an identity for himself. Therefore human beings differ in shape, size and behaviour; they also differ in the manner in which they live, love and form relationships. Therefore, love, sex, desire, passion, lust—whatever be the term—has many faces and is expressed in myriad ways.

No one knows exactly when, why and how same-sex love entered human consciousness. The fact, however, that there can be attraction between people of the same gender has been known since the dawn of humanity. The word 'eunuch', or castrated male, for example, is Greek in origin and was commonly used to refer to both homosexuals and castrated men. The term 'homosexual' itself came into use in language only in the late 19th century in Europe with the advent of modern psychiatry but this does not mean homosexuality as a sexual preference did not exist before. Sapphism or lesbianism are not contemporary constructs either; rather Sapphism draws its name from the fabled Greek lyricist Sappho who was one of the first women poets of the ancient world. Sappho, a wealthy lady born around 625 BC chose to pursue her passion for the arts living on the isle of Lesbos. There she became one of the first poets to write about love from personal experience, which in her case drew heavily from her relationships with women students who came to her to study art. The fact that Plato honoured Sappho elevating her to the status of one of the muses and that her poetry, decidedly homoerotic in content, was celebrated, could well suggest that love between women was in those times an accepted emotion. Sappho became so synonymous with love between women that two of the most definitive words in the English language to describe female homosexuality—lesbian and Sapphic—have been derived from her.

Historians claim that the earliest accounts of homosexual or Sapphic activity were part of what is today considered to be pagan rituals, and an intrinsic part of the social and religious rubric of the times. From the city-states of ancient Greece and Rome to the Siberian shamans, African tribesmen and Chinese emperors, society understood and made space for man's vulnerability to be attracted to the beauty of one's own sex. Love between males in many ways had the same standing as the marriages of the period, 'It was accepted that men did fall in love with other men, dreamt about them, wrote about them, fought over them, and took them to bed.' Nowhere is this better documented than in ancient Greece where the God of Love, Eros, was viewed equally as being heterosexual and homosexual. Male love, it was believed, brought out the best qualities in youth, especially masculinity and courage. A famous drinking song from 5th century BCE Greece declares:

Hear the four best things a man can ask of life:
Health unmarred lifelong, beauty of form and act,
Honest gain of wealth, and while one is still a boy,
To come to brightest bloom among heroic lovers.

The association of homosexual feelings with moral looseness is obviously a comparatively recent phenomenon for the Greeks equated love between men with all that was the best in human nature. Greek civilization that wholeheartedly accepted same-sex love was also responsible for evolving the concepts of democracy, philosophy, mathematics and history besides the finest theories of theatre, poetry, art and dramaturgy.

Nor was this exuberance restricted to Greece. In the 4th century, Thebes one of the largest and richest cities in central Greece saw the creation of a battalion of homosexual lovers known as the Sacred Band. In Crete there is evidence of ritualized abduction of younger boys by older men. In Japan, an apprentice Samurai pairing up with an older warrior to be trained in love and war was a common phenomenon. The samurai called it *Bi-do*, or the beautiful way, and revered the emotional and erotic bond between an older warrior and his younger apprentice. Homosexuality among the Samurais had many names, including *Nanshoku* (the love of the Samurai), *Wakashudo* (the way of the youth), *Bi-do* (the beautiful way), and *Shudo* (an abbreviation of *Wakashudo*). Even the Shogun who had numerous concubines had an equal number of young boyfriends, their 'Nanshoku' loves recorded by writers and Shunga (erotic) painters. Likewise, the hard lives of the *Tobiko*, young travelling Kabuki actors who had to labour on stage by day and please their clients in bed by night, have been immortalized in verse and prose. In Islamic Sufi literature too homosexual eroticism became a major metaphorical expression of the spiritual relationship between God and man, and much Persian poetry and fiction used gay relationships as examples of a love that was considered moral. For Arabs, so medieval travellers claim, 'Women were for home and hearth and boys were for pleasure.'

In the *Symposium*, a treatise dedicated to the issue of love and sexual pleasure, written by the Greek philosopher Plato sometime around the 5th BC, Aristophanes, one of the main characters engaged in the dialogue, offers a colorful explanation for why all these sexual options existed. According to him, 'In the beginning there were three types of double-headed humans, varying according to sex: male/male, female/female, and male/female. Zeus, angered at the humans, punished them by splitting them in half. From then on, each half has forever sought out his other half.' Which in turn led to several variations and combinations.

This is not too different from the famous books published by Dr Alfred C Kinsey called *Sexual Behaviour in the Human Male* and *Sexual Behaviour in the Human Female* based on the study of human sexuality. These studies collectively known as the Kinsey Reports indicated that there is a broad spectrum of sexual orientations that cannot be narrowed down to just heterosexual and homosexual. Instead of looking at sexual orientation as an either/or condition, Kinsey developed a seven-point continuum based on the degree of sexual responsiveness people have to members of the same and other sex. Kinsey was so struck by the extraordinary extent of individual variation in sexual behaviour that he argued that any attempt to establish uniform standards of sexual behaviour was both impracticable and unjust. He believed that the widespread deviation from accepted sexual standards showed that any attempt to regulate sexual behaviour was doomed to failure and that the only proper sexual policy was no policy at all. That the concept of sexuality and gender is only relative is best demonstrated by biology,

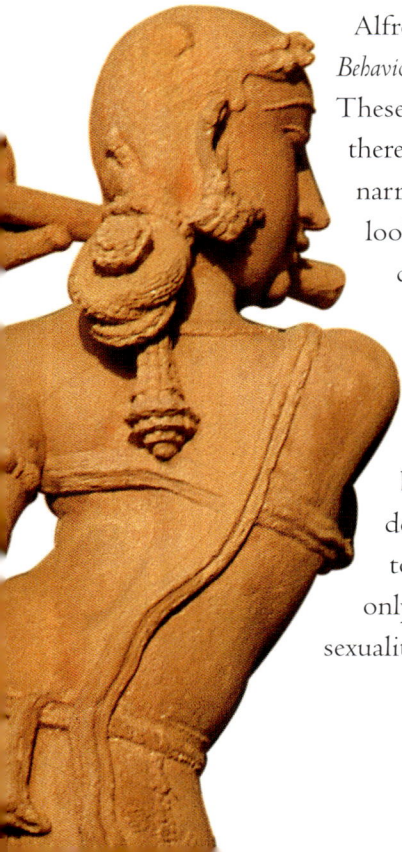

which conclusively demonstrates how among some animals males can turn into females by the mere increase of feed or temperature. In several other species sex reversals take place naturally, others go through a phase of sexual ambiguity while yet others are hermaphrodites, possessing both male and female organs. Biology-based research has even led some historians to go to the extent of believing that the early ancestors of the human race were in fact androgynous.

Vedic literature of ancient India has much to contribute towards our understanding of this important issue. Seminal works like Panini's *Ashtadhyyayi*, Bharata's *Natyashastra*, Kautilya's *Arthashastra* and Vatsyayana's *Kama Sutra* hold a great deal of relevance in today's modern society as they practically cover all facets of life ranging from right conduct, the value of education, the learning of fine arts, issues of governance and state administration, and sexuality as well. None of these works are religious but their philosophy was deeply rooted in the traditional, religious and spiritual beliefs of India. All these texts emphasize the need for knowledge and that it should be obtained through first-hand personal experience. Thus, knowledge became a personal adventure, not merely for acquiring intellectual and ego-satisfying trivia but a quest for the wisdom to influence and shape events. The pursuit to know more, the capacity to look in awe and wonder at the mysteries of the world were also transformed into an aesthetic sensibility. 'The paradox of sexual pleasure is that all those conditions which create sexual pleasure and happiness lie outside sexuality,' writes the well-known Indian historian, commentator and philosopher Badrinath Chaturvedi in his introduction to the *Kama Sutra*, thereby meaning that a

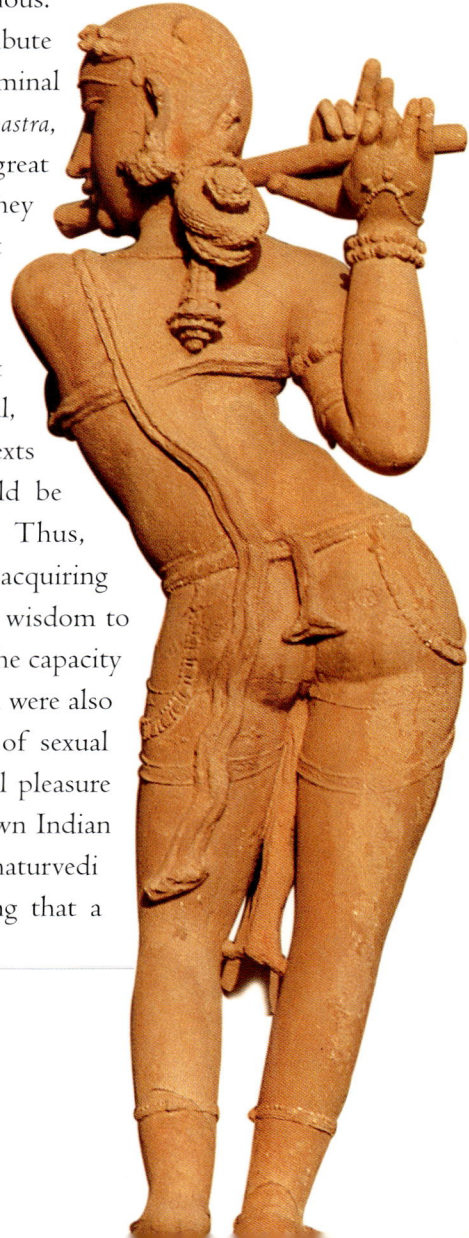

The fine art of aesthetics judiciously cultivated is a pre-requisite to understanding the nuances of sexual pleasure.

judicious cultivation of the fine art of aesthetics was a pre-requisite to understanding the nuances of sexual pleasure. Thus, to become a refined aesthete, a thorough knowledge of painting, literature, sculpture, dance and theatre was necessary and expanded the intuitive and imaginative powers of the mind.

'The distinctive Hindu concept of *svadharma* (right conduct for an individual) gives wide latitude to individuals whose gender roles and identities vary from the cultural norm. The genius of Hinduism is that it allows for so many different ways of being human,' writes Gilbert Herdt in his *Third Sex, Third Gender: Beyond Sexual Dimorphism in Culture and History*. Indian civilization thus allowed for a diversity of perceptions, lifestyles and values to the extreme and was non-judgmental almost to a fault. Yet there appears to have been a method to this madness: complex social and spiritual systems evolved which allowed for unity in diversity and made for harmonious co-existence. The amazing modernity that was exhibited from the earliest days challenges contemporary orthodoxies and attitudes towards sexual behaviour. India drew no distinctions between sacred and profane love because all love was seen as a divine mystery that had to be fully explored and experienced. Recognizing that there were people who stood outside the accepted heterosexual-marriage-children paradigm, society accepted the need for them to be respected and honoured so that they too could become successful citizens who contributed positively and significantly to thought, literature, arts and culture. The primary goal of the Hindu scriptures was to encourage and ensure all human beings, their sexual orientation notwithstanding, to pursue a spiritual life. They believed that practising the three aspects of the *purusharthas* (goals of life)—*dharma* or righteousness, *artha* or wealth, and *kama* or desire, made it possible to lead a meaningful and joyous life. The stress was on balance and integration; neglecting one of these areas would lead to diminished stability and a dangerous imbalance in men. So the ancients studied sex, practised and dissected it, classified its many methods, shared their knowledge about techniques and passed on what they had learnt. They explored not merely the physicality of intercourse but examined its pleasures and pitfalls—impotency, unequal expectations, virility and aphrodisiacs, courtesans, etiquette and manners, thus covering every conceivable aspect of society.

Born of this liberal, vibrant and modern society, the *Kama Sutra* generally acknowledged to have been compiled around the 3rd century AD, provides a window to an ancient Hindu heritage very different from the one conveyed in most philosophical and religious discourses. It gives glimpses of the social, cultural and erotic life of a people who were energetic, life affirming, tolerant and surprisingly far ahead of their times. Reinforcing attitudes towards sexuality from a bygone era, Vatsyayana's work has become a definitive manifesto of a highly evolved culture. Although viewed today as merely a manual that describes impossible sexual positions and the techniques of intercourse, the *Kama Sutra* is an expression of the vigorous sexuality found in a civilization which believed that sexual activity was almost a religious duty. Make no mistake, none of these scriptures exhorts us to pursue a life of hedonistic pleasure, rather monogamy was the norm rather than the exception, but there was acceptance of the fact that life and love had to be based on mutual respect, tolerance and faith, making it everyone's right to seek mutual sexual fulfillment.

The pragmatic Vatsyayana therefore explores aspects of adultery and acknowledges the fact that men although married would continue to pursue other women. The *Kama Sutra* goes into great detail about the process of the seduction of the *parkiya* or women who are not one's own. In keeping with the social milieu of the time, *ganikas* or courtesans were a respected and accepted part of life as were temporary relationships, contractual arrangements, relationships with housemaids, and pleasure houses populated by women trained in the art and craft of love. Neither are other aspects of sexuality ignored— homosexuals, lesbians, prostitutes and eunuchs or persons of the 'third nature', were all included. In *Like a City Ablaze: The Third Sex and the Creation of Sexuality in Jain Religious Literature,* Michael Sweet and Leonard Zwilling observe that various sexually ambiguous categories, 'have been a part of the Indian worldview for nearly three thousand years'. All variants thus had a place and position as was illustrated by the sociological and moral texts of Vedic India which accepted, much like the Kinsey Reports variations on three basic kinds of natures *(prakrtis)* or genders in society, namely the *pums-prakrti* or men, *striya-prakrti* or women, and the *tritiya-prakrti* or the third gender. Contrary to the modern notion of homosexuality that is defined as a preference for a partner of the same sex, homosexuality in ancient India was not determined by physical characteristics alone, but by an assessment of the entire being that includes the gross (physical) body, the subtle (psychological) body, and a unique consideration based upon social interaction or procreative status. In ancient erotic and medical texts, male as well as female homosexuals were thus part of a group belonging to the 'third nature' (*tritiya prakrti*), characterized by the lack of procreative ability or the will to procreate, and consisted among others of gay males, *svairinis* or lesbians, eunuchs, women who were barren.

The idea of human beings who are not quite male or female was known in India for a long time. Such people were known as *kliba*, a word that included a wide range of meanings under the general rubric of 'a man who does not act the way a man should act,' a man lacking in heterosexual desire, a man who had sex with other men, etc. Bisexual women known as *kamini*s were known to entice men and enjoy sex to their full satisfaction. Lesbians or *svairini*s were independent or liberated women who refused to marry, earned their own livelihood and lived either alone or in marriage with one of their own kind. And then there were the *stri rajyas*, states and communities that were entirely ruled by women. Strong lesbian feelings and activities are known to have existed in such female kingdoms during

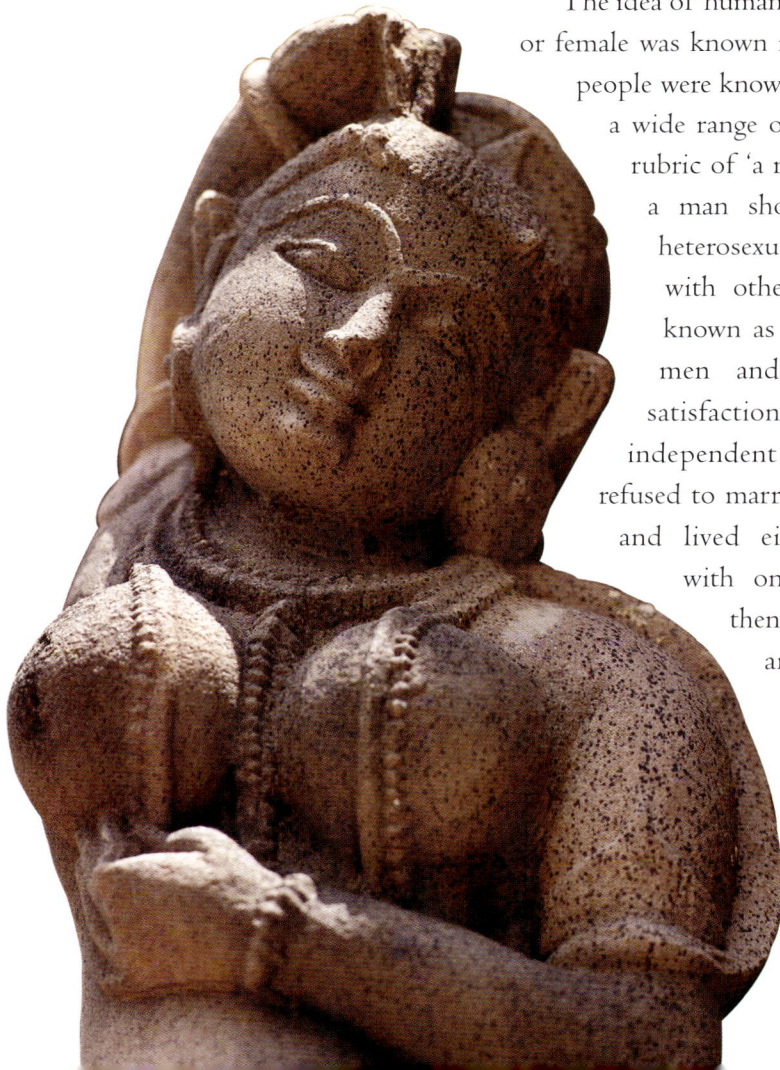

the latter part of the 1st century, when repeated wars left societies bereft of men. References to female kingdoms abound in Kautilya's *Arthashastra*, in the *Mahabharata*, as well as in the travelogues of Hiuen Tsang, the 7th century Chinese pilgrim. Vatsyayana in the *Kama Sutra* also describes these 'matriarchal countries' as places where 'brutal sexual behaviour are required' to satisfy women, where 'dildos are much employed', and where women often hide young men in their apartments for sexual use. People who fell into this third category were invariably recognized as being proficient in the arts, with a fine cultivated sense of aesthetics, good entertainers, exceptional musicians, dancers, beauticians, hair dressers, cooks and domestic help. They were also considered to be auspicious and their blessings much sought after at wedding ceremonies.

The *Kama Sutra* was not a one-off aberration, for between the 10th and 17th centuries, several texts similar to the *Kama Sutra* were written, most of them by noblemen and kings, who refined the art of lovemaking. One such text the *Manmata Samhita*, which in fact is a paean to the month of spring, exhorts everyone to seek their pleasure and explore their sexuality in whatever form available. The *Manmata Samhita* eulogizes passion from which no one is excluded—young girls, boys, older women, widows, eunuchs, people of the third gender, young married couples, just about everyone is advised to seek sexual satisfaction, 'for not experiencing passion during the month of spring is tantamount to sin'. So whatever be the form gender or desire took, balance and harmony constituted the touchstone of Indian philosophy, and men and women were encouraged to wholeheartedly explore their quest for sexual fulfillment. These centuries-old teachings encouraged intercourse not merely for procreation but for pleasure and intimacy, as well as for lifelong health, creativity, and longevity.

Nor was the acceptance of same-sex love restricted to Hindu sensibilities. Buddhist scriptures or the Pali canon, for example, also contain references to homosexuality among monks. The Pali equivalent word for the Hindu *kliba* is

Facing page: Whatever form gender or desire takes, balance and harmony constitute the touchstone for happiness.

pandaka. Like Hinduism, Buddhism too eschews all kinds of sexual behaviour that require subterfuge and deceit, where vows are broken and there is a betrayal of trust. Unlike Hindu social codes where marriage and the raising of children are seen as compulsory, forming the bedrock of social life, Buddhism places no particular value on procreation. Instead celibacy is considered to be a requirement for those seeking higher levels of development. 'Buddhism contains numerous references to sexual behaviour that today would be identified as homoerotic and to individuals who would be called homosexual and transvestites,' writes Peter A Jackson in his essay, 'Non normative Sex/Gender Categories in Theravada Buddhist Scriptures.' According to him, 'The Pali canon does not clearly distinguish between homosexuality from cross-gender behaviour such as transvestitism and male-male sex is referred to in many places in the *Vinayapitaka*.' He makes a reference to the *Buddhaghosa* which describes hermaphroditism as arising from a dissonance between the masculine and feminine 'power' *(indriya)* of an individual and their sexual organs *(byanjana).* In Buddhism as in Hinduism, however, all forms of sexuality and desire had to be acknowledged and transcended in order to attain nirvana or moksha.

The forms of love and courtship vary with each culture and the forces that shape human behaviour are no longer instinctive but are formed by cultivated habits which in turn have been shaped by factors like education, upbringing and tradition. There is a growing realization today, a fact very clearly recognized by the wise sage Vatsyayana, that there can be and is an astonishing variety of patterns that fall within a basic social and moral construct. The world now celebrates with a great deal of enthusiasm the so-called sexual revolution. But this rebellion appears to have stemmed more from social disobedience rather than a real quest for freedom of expression. Sexual freedom or self-expression only comes with responsibility, which in turn requires maturity, understanding and development of the whole person, or as Hindu theology demands—a spiritual life.

The same held true of Tantra. The quest for ecstasy—the search for meaning,

Facing page: In Tantra every sexual practice conceivable is practised and venerated in an attempt to transcend the senses through the senses.

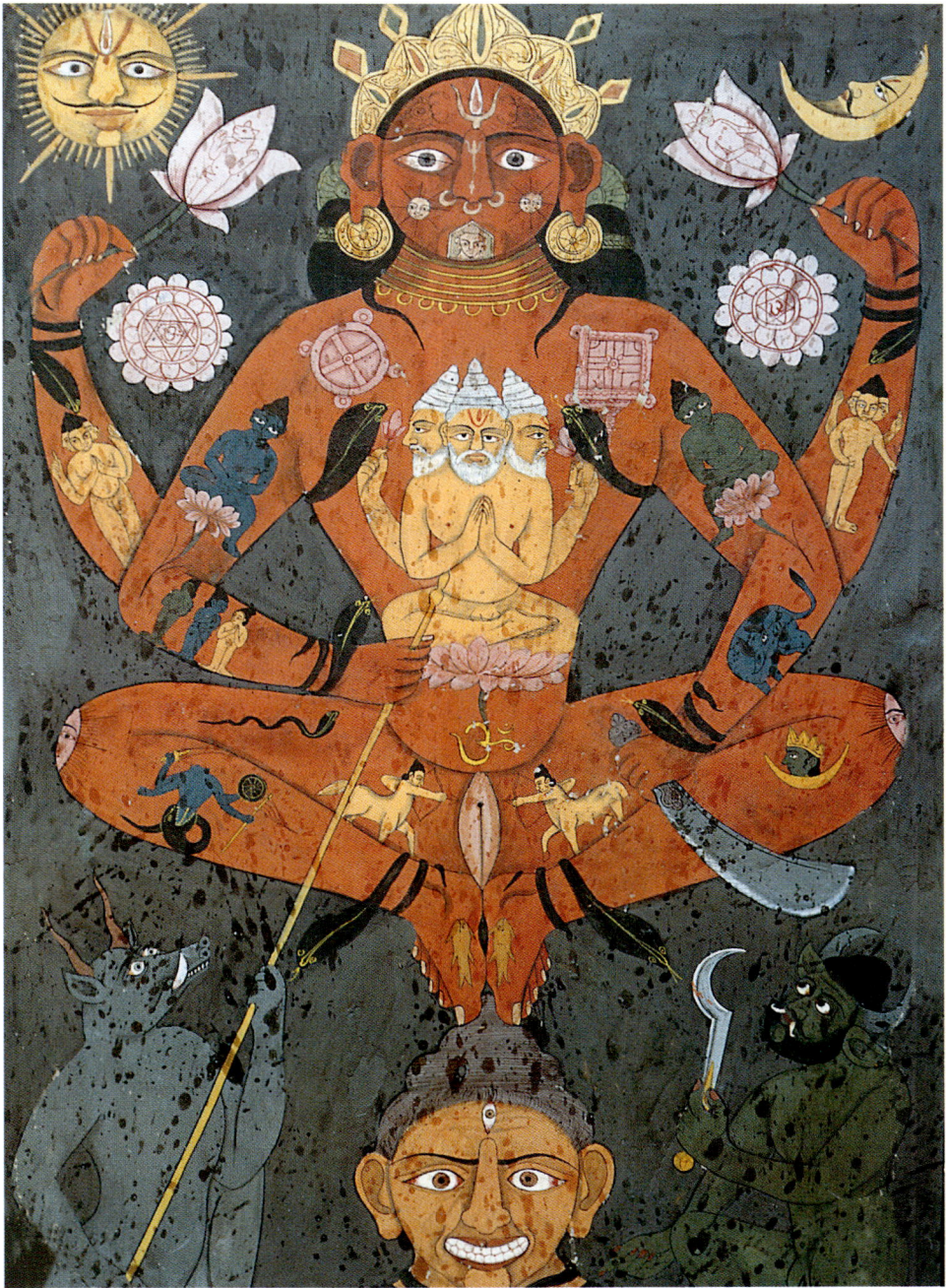

pleasure, and lasting bliss—has been an important current in all human history, and dates back much before the '60s flower power revolution. Although the historicity of Tantra is difficult to determine, some scholars believe it to have been a pre-Aryan practice existing as far back as 3000 BC. Tantra propounded the belief that sex was a means to spiritual advancement. Subsequently based on the deities that became associated with many Tantric cults, emerged the Shaiva, Shakti and Kaula cults, their traditions, rituals and forms of worship setting them apart from existing religious traditions. In Tantra's evolution, almost every sexual practice conceivable was practised and venerated in an attempt to transcend the senses through the senses. An orgasm was seen as a release of personal vices, a liberation of the ego and thought, a way to transcend rational consciousness, a moment when one could experience oneness with a divine Higher Being. Seen thus, Tantra did not make a moral issue of sex, whatever form it took.

Tantra, however, is not a religion, but a mystical and philosophical dimension, much like the Jewish Kabbala, that stresses the need for firsthand experience, and the experiential nature of a practice rather than blind adherence to any belief or dogma. Tantra strives to inculcate a new level of mastery over one's body, to heal emotional scars, and explore the intimate relationship between spirituality and sexuality. Tantrics claim that it is the most original and easiest path to salvation and devised techniques of prolonging an orgasm in order to experience first hand God or Consciousness. Tantra, like Hinduism ultimately is of the belief that all Reality is one, that the duality we perceive, especially the sexual duality of the separateness of man and woman, is at the heart of anxieties and unhappiness. Tantra is about transcending this duality and seeking the one reality that encompasses all diversity. Thus while ancient India accepted that pleasure was primary it advocated that the pursuit of pleasure should always be tempered with sensitivity, common sense, reverence for life, tolerance, consideration for others and most importantly control over oneself. Thus hedonism, if it was that, was ethical and combined sexuality with civility, closely interlinking morality and social behaviour. Eroticism was valued but not when it infringed upon the rights of others.

Juxtaposed against the seemingly more cultivated Western liberal humanism, ancient India's openness towards all things sexual may appear idyllic, almost overt. But every philosophical tenet around the world maintains that seeking fulfillment is the purpose and programme of human existence. Although modern society believes that moral values must be derived from experience, and ethics should stem from human needs and interest, the world appears to have lost much of its past tolerance for multiplicity as well as its appreciation of diversity.

Modern liberalism continues to suffer from unresolved contradictions and inbuilt hypocrisies even as society slips into excesses like rape, violence and abuse. Intolerance towards sexuality is often cultivated by orthodox religions and puritanical cultures that continue to repress it, often finding its way into even political platforms. The right to birth control, abortion, and same-sex marriages are still debated hotly with no resolution in sight; the many varieties of sexual exploration are still perceived as running counter to prevailing religious beliefs. Many traditional religions continue to reject the scientific, medical and psychological knowledge that we have gained about sexuality and regard homosexuality as a 'choice' or a 'moral evil', thereby if anything, causing more division, hatred, bigotry, violence and oppression. There are the radicals who set gays apart as a new breed within society and there are those who would like to see gays assimilated into mainstream society with the only difference being same-sex behaviour. No wonder gays around the world are rejecting religion for politics making it imperative for these rigid and fundamentalist regimes to discuss and analyse topics that were once declared as taboo.

Superimposing morality and sexual restraint on a society only leads to rebellion for people perceive moral laws as policing that forces them to adopt stringent standards of conduct that are not natural. Sexual restraint such as monogamy or celibacy was only effective when voluntary. To explore one's potential free from fear, self-consciousness and inhibition, is a fundamental right of mankind. Understanding is required to enhance our worldview. Without countenancing mindless permissiveness or unbridled promiscuity, a civilized society should be a tolerant one. Short of harming or coercing individuals, they should be permitted to express their sexual proclivities and pursue their lifestyles as they desire. Society

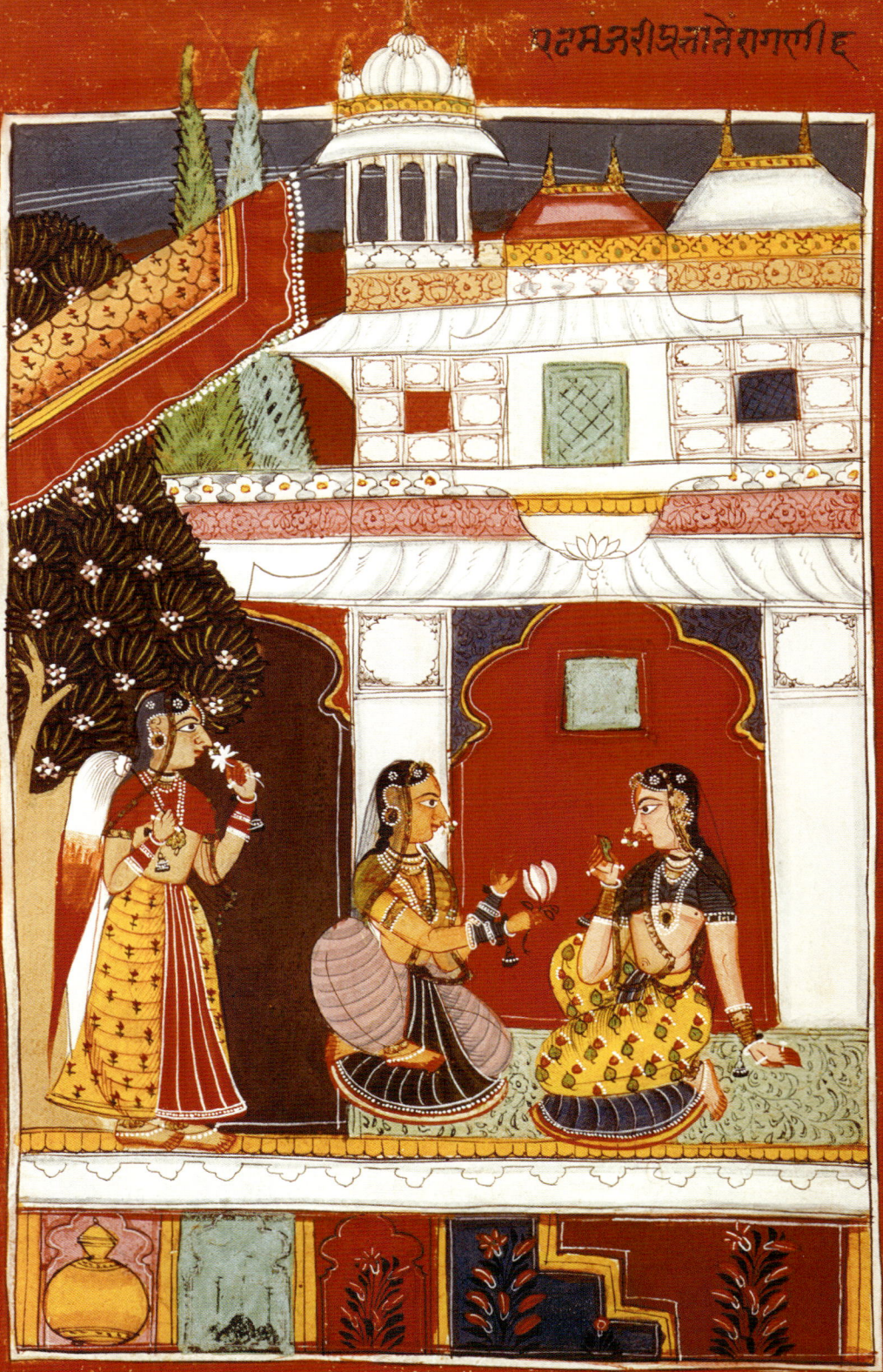

needs to cultivate a responsible attitude toward sexuality, in which humans are not exploited as sexual objects and in which intimacy, sensitivity, respect and honesty in interpersonal relations are encouraged.

This can come from studying and understanding texts like the *Kama Sutra* which enables us to shed our misconceptions and prejudices. Clearly debunking modern arguments that sexual information leads to decadence and perversion, this text inspires men and women who chose to live by their own sexual proclivities, with its openness and adaptability. By adapting ancient techniques, positions that are unlimited in their exciting variations and urbane wisdom, it enables them to explore the full range of human passion. More than anything else, the *Kama Sutra* encourages holistic living. Be it through the diverse methods of foreplay and various positions that make intercourse pleasurable, the interplay between people who were sexually ambivalent, the acceptance without rancour into society of people of the third sex, the extensive use of *aupanisadika* or special appliances as aids, the various methods of using aphrodisiacs, or the concepts of Tantra, there is much to learn from the *Kama Sutra*. Although pleasure is at the heart of this text, the larger lesson that this ancient text teaches us is one of balance, tolerance and sensitivity, for only after fully understanding these basic tenets can people begin their quest to realize their full potential as human beings.

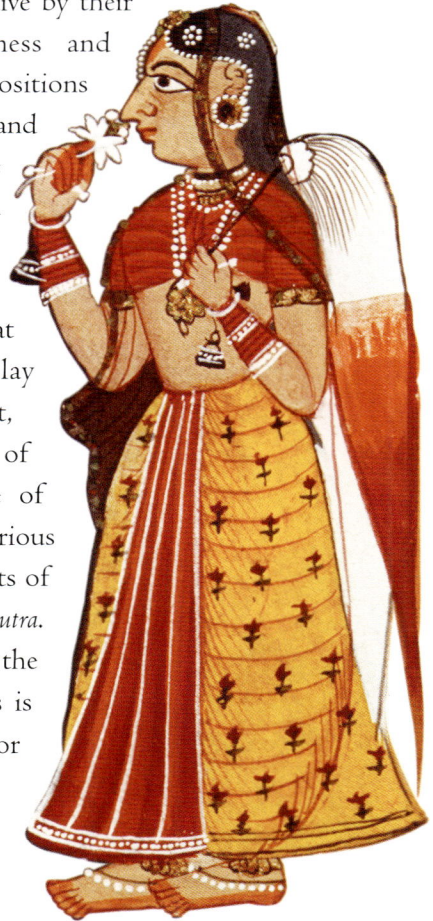

Facing page: Although pleasure is at the heart of every sexual experience, the larger quest is to realize one's full potential as a human being.

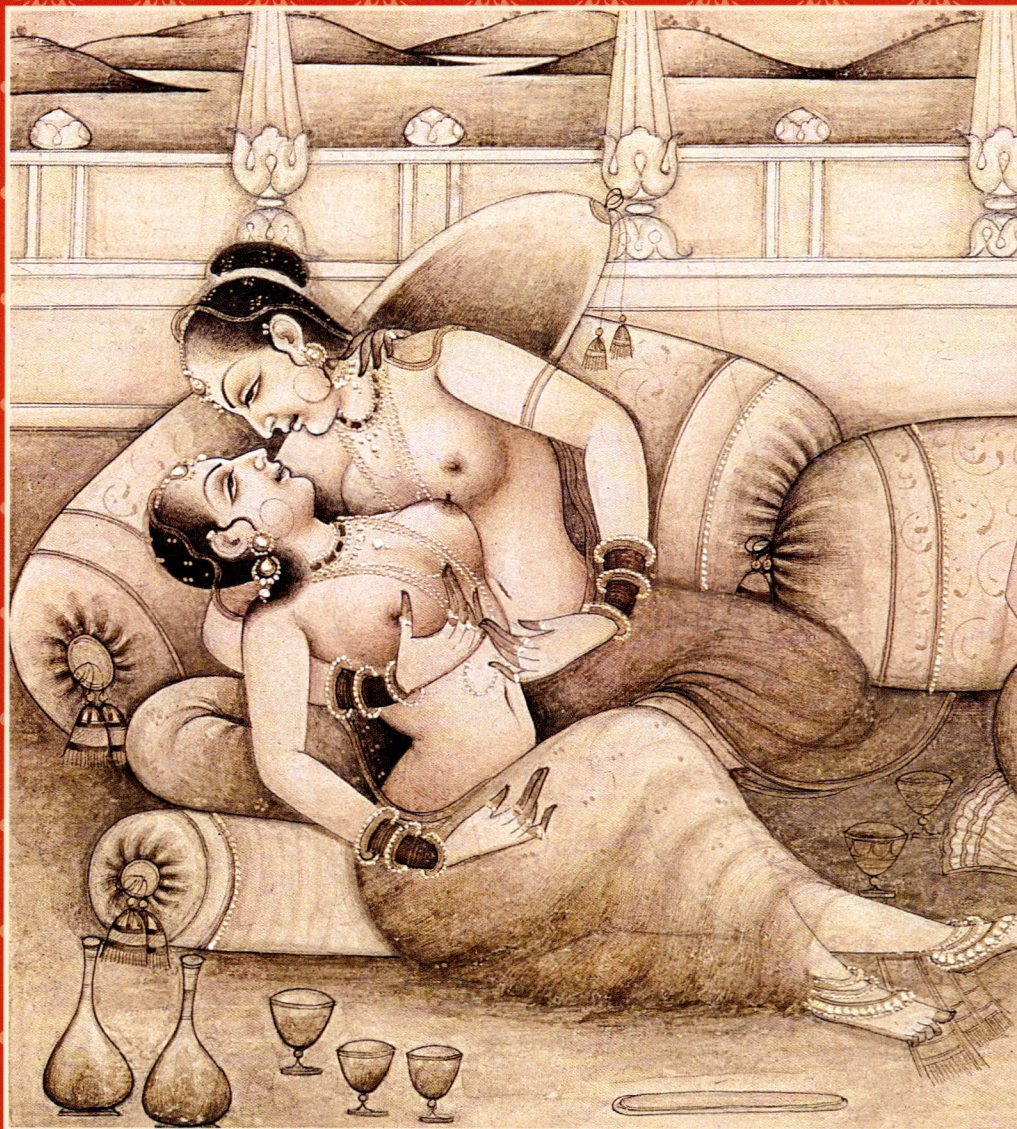

Gay mythologies

From the earliest times, as men have sought to understand and relate to the inscrutability of the universe, myths have supplied a sense of meaning and direction to help transcend mundane existence and give significance to life. Unravelling a world of mystery and awe, mythologies have also given the universe a spiritual hue—painting 'a holy picture', as it were. These vivid, often erotic attempts to explain the inexplicable and unknown to the modern mind, may often seem fanciful or bizarre, but narrated as tales and poetry, ballads and drama, they have become mythologies that have endured.

From the earliest times mythologies were used to explain creation and the genesis of the gods, more often than not, using sexual metaphors. From the cave people who illustrated their caves with graphic erotic drawings of pregnant women worshipped for their fecundity, to the various cultures that existed in the Middle East like Mesopotamia where Ishtar was the Babylonian goddess of love, fertility, nature and sex, the Pheonicians, Amorites, Canaanites, Hitties, Philistines, and ancient Egypt that displayed divergent sexual behaviour like homosexuality, trans-genderism, incest marriages, exhibitionism, prostitution, adultery, bestiality, necrophilia, among others, the spread of myth narration has been a universal phenomenon. Ancient cultures like India and China told their tales in vivid sexual imagery as did the ancient Greeks for whom Zeus's penis became the womb for the gods. The Incas, Aztecs and Mayans too had their own creation mythologies. These erotic mythologies continue to exist in every culture and religious tradition as a means of explaining human fecundity, fertility in nature or as a means of appeasing the gods. 'All over the world and at different times of human history, these archetypes, or elementary ideas, have appeared in different costumes. The differences in the costumes are the results of environment and historical conditions,' said the late Joseph Campbell, the world's leading expert on mythology.

To ancient pagan thinkers, as well as to modern psychologists, the key to the hidden secret of the origin and preservation of the universe lies hidden in the mysteries of sex and gender. Viewed from any perspective, it was the coming together of the male generative power and the feminine aspect that resulted in life. These opposing but complementary energies found representation in a number of eastern philosophies oftentimes assuming anthropomorphic forms and becoming closely associated with fertility, agriculture and war. These gods were thus never gender specific, could be both, or male/female, were fallible and often like ordinary people, had physical desires. Almost all mythologies believed that gods too had sex and procreated. The most persistent example of this is what is known as *Hieros Gamos* or sacred marriage where either symbolically or through actual sex, a deity mates with a human ritualist, or two deities mate with each other to encourage crops to grow. At least once a year in ancient societies that were based on agriculture, people dressed as gods, and engaged in sexual intercourse to guarantee the fertility of the land. The festival began with a procession, followed by an exchange of gifts, a purification rite, the wedding feast, the preparation of the wedding chamber, and a secret nocturnal act of intercourse. Other practices confirm that the wrath of the gods could be appeased or salvation could be obtained by ritualized sacrifices which in some cases like Tantra, translated into having sex with another as part of the process of worship itself. This certainly raised no eyebrows especially if help was being sought, amidst other things, for a good monsoon, fertile crops, healthy cattle, and healthy children.

In his interesting essay titled 'Homosexuality in History', Reverend Robert J. Buchanan writes: 'Homosexual practices may have become a part of polytheistic worship as a successor to masturbation. If one believed that having sex with a god would bring fertility, it was easy to also believe that, if a man added his maleness, through his semen, to a male god, fertility would be multiplied all the more. When a man ejaculated his semen into another man's anus at the shrine, he was depositing more male power to the gods. With the additional strength of many men, the god could then insure a bountiful crop, a larger herd, and many children to care for the field.' This practice, according to Reverend Buchanan, grew into not only forms of pagan worship, but also a means of supplying money for the temple. Catamites or boys and men who were exclusively used for passive anal sex, began to serve the temples.

Some legends are indeed more explicit and overt than others. For example, the main god of the Phoenicians was known as Asshur or Asher, meaning the penis—the happy one. Another of their gods was Dagon, represented as half-fish and half-man; the fish being worshipped as a fertility symbol from the earliest times because of the female fish's ability to lay thousands of eggs. The Sumerians too had their own creation myth in which the god Ninmah fashioned seven variations of human beings including a category of 'one who has no male organ, no female organ' and a 'woman who cannot give birth'. Similarly in the Akkadian myth of Atrahasis (*ca.* 1700 BCE), the god Enki instructs Nintu, the Goddess of Birth, to establish a 'third category among the people' that includes demons who steal infants, women who are unable to give birth, and priestesses who are prohibited from bearing children. Much in the same manner, the early Babylonians too had a god called Baal who was often worshipped as a phallic symbol. Many of the Babylonian cities erected towers or ziggurats that were used variously as observation posts, defense points, as well as shrines. Early worship at these towers included masturbation, allowing the man to spill his semen on the earth which was seen as female.

An extreme case was that of Egypt whose religion was very complex because of its polytheistic pantheon. According to Egyptian legend, Amun or Amon was the First Being who is often depicted as a well-built man wearing a crown depicting the head of a ram. In the beginning Amun existed alone before the creation of the universe but created the universe sexually by drinking his own semen and thus impregnating himself. The other main god was Osiris, initially a corn god who became the symbol of the generative power of nature sometimes depicted with three phalloi. The worship of the Apis bull was also part of the Egyptians' sacred rites and the French traveller Vivant Denon speaks of the finding of the embalmed phallus of a bull interred with a female mummy. Sexuality in Egypt was thus open, untainted by guilt and accepted as an important aspect of life. Interestingly the Egyptians even believed in sex in the afterlife so Egyptian mythologies are replete with tales of adultery, incest, homosexuality and masturbation, with hints of necrophilia. Tales of homosexuality between gods also abound illustrated by the tale of Set, one of ancient Egypt's earliest gods and Horus, the child of the godess Isis and Orisis. Set said to Horus, 'Come, let us have a feast day at my house.' And Horus said to him, 'I will, I will.' Now when evening had come, a bed was prepared for them, and they lay down together. At night, Set let his member become stiff, and he inserted it between the thighs of Horus. And Horus placed his hand between his thighs and caught the semen of Set.

Nowhere is eroticism especially homosexuality so celebrated as in Greece, a fact that is conspicuously exhibited in every aspect of life in its ancient times. Greek sculpture as well as its pottery and paintings for example are highly erotic: satyrs and nymphs cavort naked under olive trees, young men and women are seen bathing, dancing, and making love. If these paintings are to be believed, the Greeks even fought their battles either naked or nearly so and found nothing strange about that. The Greek pantheon too was made of gods who were extremely volatile, emotional and sensuous. Zeus, the King of the Gods, whose origins can be traced back to the Indian Dyaus pitar (the creator god mentioned in the *Ŗg Veda*) is credited with what was even then known as Greek love or homosexuality. Legend has it that a Trojan prince called Ganymede was famous as the most handsome of men on earth. One day when Ganymede was bathing in the Mediterranean, Zeus happened to catch a glimpse of the young Trojan's thighs which instantly aroused the god's passions. Disregarding Hera, Zeus's wife who fumed in silence, the god took the shape of an eagle, abducted the handsome prince and carried him off to Mount Olympus. There the two men romped around loving each other. Zeus, because he liked the boy's kisses best, made him immortal and set the young man among the stars as Aquarius.

The other Greek man celebrated for his heroism and prowess in the battlefield and bed was of course Hercules. Strong and wise, he is credited with having made love to the forty-nine virgin daughters of a king named Thespios. Much as he loved women, Hercules loved young boys too; numerous were his lovers including several young Argonauts like Admetos, Iphitos, and Euphemos. Legend also has it that Eurystheus, the king for whom Hercules performed his labours, was one of his lovers. But of his many lovers, the one he loved best was his sixteen-year-old nephew called Iolaos. As the historian Plutarch who accompanied Alexander on several of his campaigns tells us: 'As to the [male] loves of Hercules, it is difficult to record them because of their number... . It is a tradition that Iolaos, who assisted Hercules in his labours and fought at his side, was beloved of him; and Aristotle observes that even in his time, lovers pledged their faith at Iolaos' tomb.'

Renowned equally for his almost superhuman military exploits as well as his devotion to his male friends and companions was Alexander the Great. The quintessential product of a patriarchal warrior culture, he epitomized male values in a world that was dominated by masculine sensibilities. His tutor from the age of seven was the philosopher Aristotle, who documented the excesses as well as the values of pederasty. Alexander went on to embody his famous tutor's values by living out his great romance with his childhood friend Hephaiston. The other great love of Alexander's life was the eunuch Bagoas, a dancer, musician and favourite of

King Darius of Persia. The friendship that grew between them was to last the rest of their lives.

The Greeks believed that the power of love experienced between men brought out the best in them, motivated them and gave them a refined sense of aesthetics. The Romans were not far behind in their belief. Pan, otherwise known as Priapus, was the fructifying god of the ancient Romans, giving rise to an epithet that found its way into modern vocabulary—priapism. Images of Pan were placed in temples and played an important part of ceremonial worship in which young girls and brides in particular had to take part the night before they were married.

Homoerotic mythologies were not confined only to the Western world. Confucius is credited with having said *'Shi se xing ye'* (food and sexuality are natural urges) which exemplifies Chinese attitudes towards sexuality. Mythological stories, heterosexual or homosexual, embody the old Chinese concepts of *P'o* and *Hun*, (two elements of the spirit—the *anima* and *animus*) as well as ancient beliefs in animal worship, the reincarnation and karmic retribution of Buddhism, and the Taoist thoughts on sexual power (*qi*, or energy flow of the human body). Believing that all events are predestined according to the deeds in one's past life, the Chinese, like the Hindus, accepted all aspects of their present, including homosexuality, as a result of their past lives. In some of the mythological stories, for example, a ghost, a fox fairy in a male body form, or even a man may perform homosexual intercourse with another living male, just because the former was his female lover in the past life. While many of the animal fairies in Chinese mythology enjoy homosexual relationships with younger men or boys, only the dragon, a symbol of the rainbow in ancient China, consistently enjoys sexual relationships with older men.

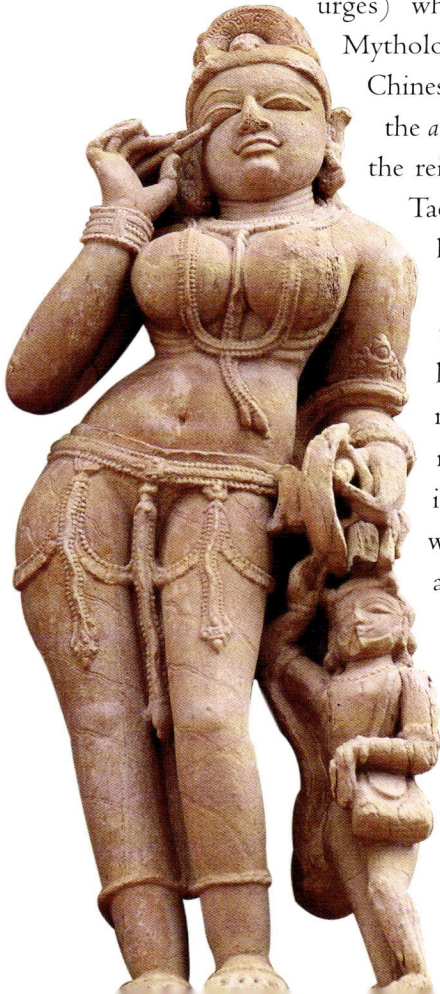

Homosexuality has been celebrated in mythologies across the world.

If Western mythologies celebrated same-sex love and believed that it brought out the best in men, the ancient Hindus adopted a more laid-back attitude towards homosexuality. The Hindus placed a great deal of importance on balance and holistic living with all aspects of life, including pleasure and desire having their own governing principles. In an attempt to understand creation and find appropriate imagery to explain it, Hindu mythology contains many stories where miraculous sexual transformation allows homoerotic desire in both men and women to be enacted. In addition there are androgynous gods and goddesses, spontaneous sexual transformations, men giving birth thereby belying the absoluteness of heterosexual relationships and static gender paradigms. Acceptance also made it possible for all forms of sexuality to become overt and organized as is corroborated by Indian literature, sculpture, painting and poetry.

The best known of all the Hindu transgendered deities is Mohini, the female incarnation of the great preserver-god Vishnu, one of the Trinity of the Hindu pantheon. Several myths on Mohini revolve around her seducing other men. In one tale, Brahma, the Lord of the Gods, tells the *devas* (minor gods) that they can obtain *amrit* or nectar by churning the divine ocean. To do this, they decide to stir it with a mountain and enlist the help of the *asuras* or demons. After several adventures, the ocean finally surrenders the nectar that they sought and at once fights break out between the gods and demons. Then, it is said, Vishnu assumes the guise of Mohini the Enchantress, and successfully distracts and seduces the *asuras* and distributes the divine nectar to the gods.

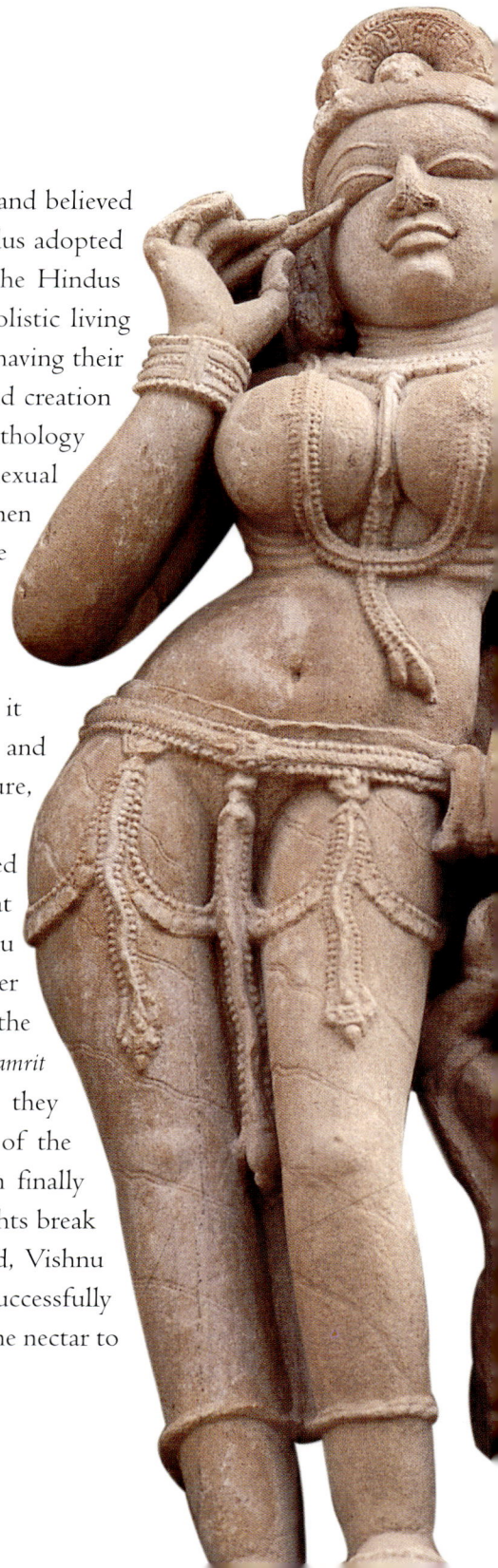

In a parallel story Vishnu transforms into the beauteous Mohini in order to save Lord Shiva, the second god of the Hindu Trinity, from Bhasmasura. By performing severe ascetic sacrifices Bhasmasura, a vile demon, is granted a boon by Shiva which empowers him to turn anyone he touches on the head into ash. Whereupon the demon attacks Shiva himself! Shiva convinces Vishnu to intervene, and Vishnu assumes the form of Mohini. Bhasmasura gets completely besotted with Mohini, who convinces him to mimic every move she makes during an alluring dance. Bhasmasura is so distracted by her beauty and grace that she tricks him into patting himself on the head thereby turning himself into ash. Shiva, while being fully aware that Mohini is none other than Vishnu is so attracted to her, that despite his wife Parvati looking on, succumbs to her charms and allows himself to be seduced by her. The result of this union is said to be Hariharaputra, a name derived from the titles of Vishnu (Hari) and Shiva (Hara). Hariharaputra is also known as Ayyappan, the hermaphrodite offspring of Mohini and Shiva.

Eunuchs or people of the third sex were not only known to ancient Indians but find prominent place in their mythology. The legend of Amba plays a pivotal role in India's best-known epic the *Mahabharata*. Amba, a young beautiful princess wants to marry the king of Salwa and she solicits the assistance

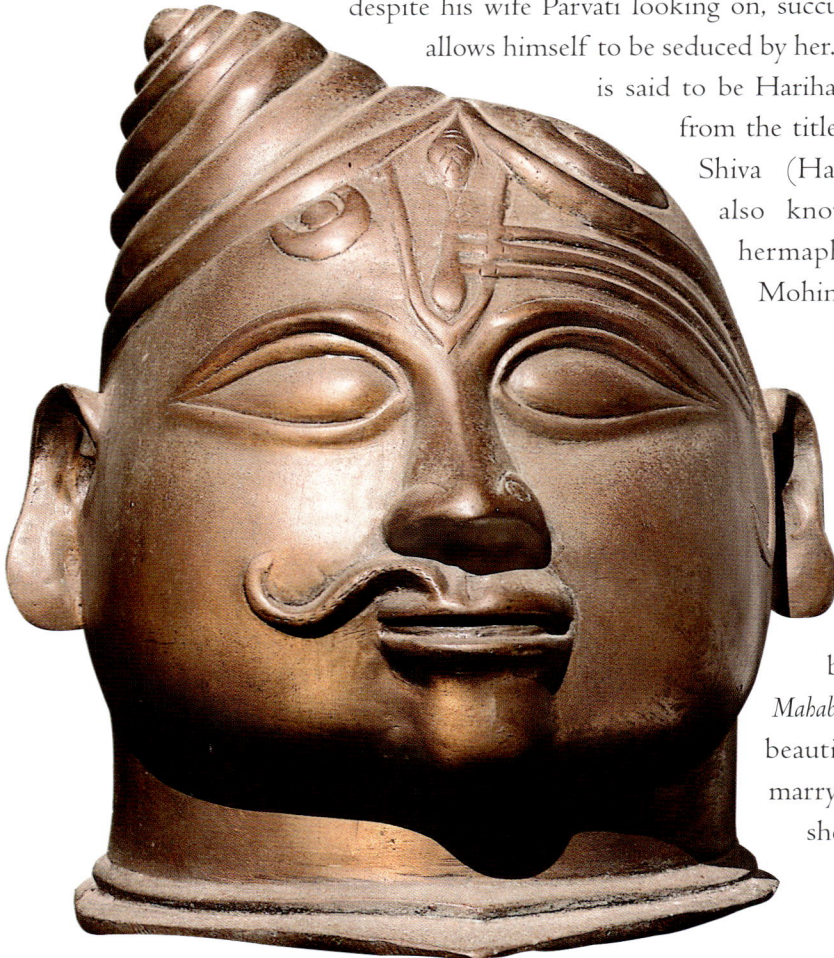

of the court elder Bhishma, to send her to the king, who unfortunately refuses to marry her. She then turns to Bhishma himself and seeks his hand in marriage, but bound by his vows of celibacy, Bhisma also rejects her offer. A dejected Amba throws herself into fire and kills herself vowing to seek revenge on Bhishma. In her next birth she is born as Shikhandi, a hermaphrodite or eunuch—of indeterminable gender. Bhishma comes face to face with her in the great battlefield of Kurukshetra. But unable to kill a human being who is sexually ambiguous, he lays down his arms and is killed in turn.

A society can be judged by the manner in which it treats its minorities. Since Vedic society was advanced culturally, it offered protection as well as a place in society to citizens of the second and third genders. The perfect example of this again can be found in the epic, the *Mahabharata* where King Virata offers both friendship and protection to Arjuna who seeks sanctuary in his court as a transgender male. King Virata, the Ruler of the Matsya province in India gives asylum to the five exiled Pandava princes. When Arjuna, one of the five brothers approaches the king for shelter, he is in the guise of Brihanalla. Arjuna introduces himself at court thus, 'Know me, O King of men to be Brihanalla, a son or daughter, without a father or mother.'

Dressed in a woman's blouse and draped in red silk with numerous ivory bangles, golden earrings and necklaces made of coral and pearls, his long hair braided, Arjuna enters the royal palace as a professional dancer and musician adept in singing, with hair decoration and 'all the fine arts that a woman should know'.

After exhibiting his skills, Arjuna is tested by beautiful women to ensure that he is indeed of the third sex and thus free from any lust for females. The king is pleased with Arjuna's manner and arranges for him to live among the palace women and educate them in singing and dancing. Arjuna in the guise of Brihanalla was treated with due respect and honoured for his skills and given

Society in Vedic India was mature culturally and offered protection as well as a place in society to citizens of all genders.

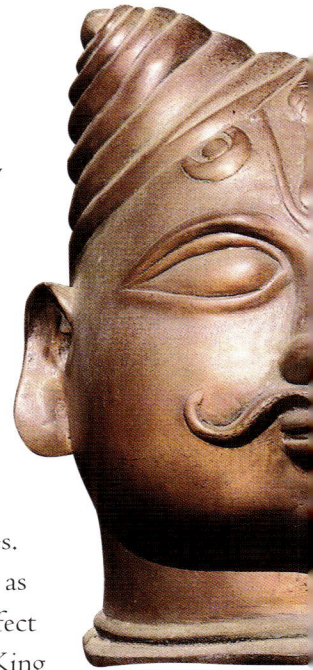

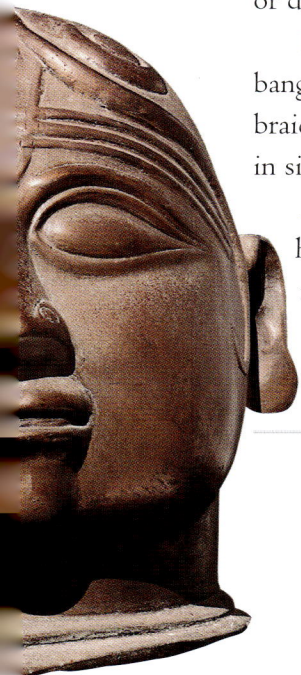

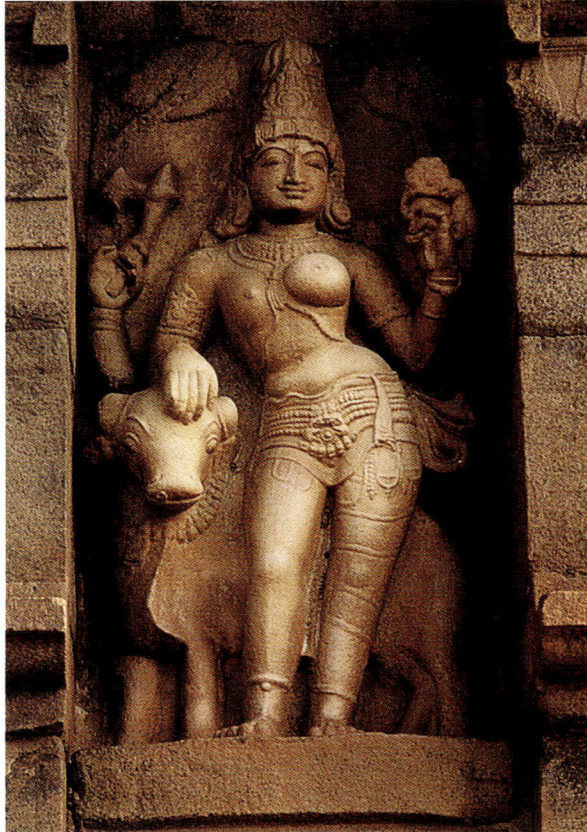

shelter and employment in the royal palace, without being ridiculed or scorned at. It would appear that from then on in most courts, feminine gay males were often professionally employed in palace harems and by aristocratic women as they were known to be proficient in the arts, entertainment and most notably in dancing. Their presence at marriage, births and other religious ceremonies was considered to be auspicious; their blessings were much sought after—a tradition that persists to this day.

The two aspects of the cosmos—the male and female that made all life on earth possible—come together in the concept of the Ardhanarishwara.

The bedrock on which Hindu philosophy rests is that of *karma*, the impact of past actions on present lives. This catch-all phrase makes it possible for ordinary Indians even today to philosophically accept what one cannot change. The emphasis was thus on acceptance, and along with other things, the average Hindu was conditioned to accept the body and sexuality as natural aspects of the cycle of birth and death. The two aspects of the cosmos—the male and the female that made all life on earth possible, finds pride of place in Hindu mythology as the *Ardhanarishwara* (half-male, half-female).

Hinduism is broadly divided into three basic schools known as Shakta, Shaiva and Vaishnava cults. In the first two the Ultimate Reality is conceived as the Unity of Shakti (the Divine Feminine) and Shiva (the Divine Masculine) thereby making the godhead androgynous or half-male and half-female. According to Hinduism, as long as sexuality and identity are based on separateness, there will always be a longing for completion; for this separation and sense of duality always results in pain and unhappiness. The androgyne, thus, reunites the separated halves into a single, complete being. The Hindu deity Ardhanarishwara is the product of just such a coupling between Shiva and Parvati, much as the Greek god Hermaphroditus is the result of his merger with the over-sexed nymph Salmicis. The Chinese *yin* and *yang* design is the perfect symbol of this form of androgyny. Typically depicted as sensuous and passive figures, they represent the release of tension between men and women, thus creating harmony and balance.

The frank sexuality of the ancient Indians, as with the other civilizations, an expression of their attempts to understand the universe, became closely associated with the worship of fertility that, eschewing morality, provided for rather exuberant outbursts of erotic expression. The unabashed honesty of the nudity that embellishes so many Hindu temples for example divested the body of any crudeness and raised it to a divine plane as well as a fine art. The entire range of sexual expressions are depicted on these temple walls: coy glances, wild orgies involving kings, queens, warriors, sages, slaves, animals, and sometimes even gods. There are no rules here—elephants are shown copulating with tigers, monkeys

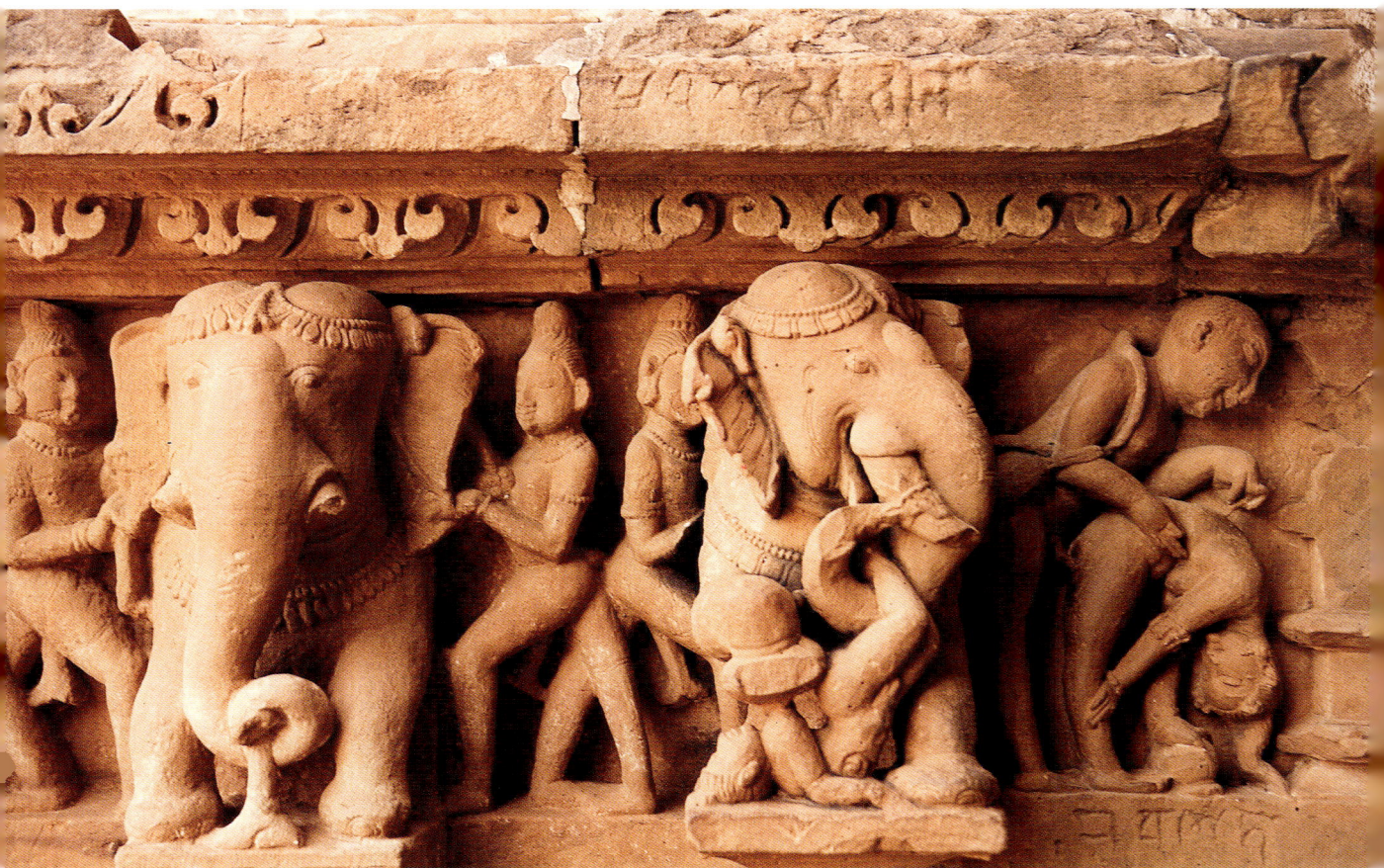

molest women while men mate with asses—and yes even images of men mating with men and women fondling each other. Such a liberated society could not ever have seen homosexuality as unnatural. Curiously enough, the cave temples of monastic orders such as Buddhism and Jainism built around the same time also have similar images embellishing prayer halls.

The frank sexuality of ancient India is closely associated with the worship of fertility, divesting the body of any crudeness.

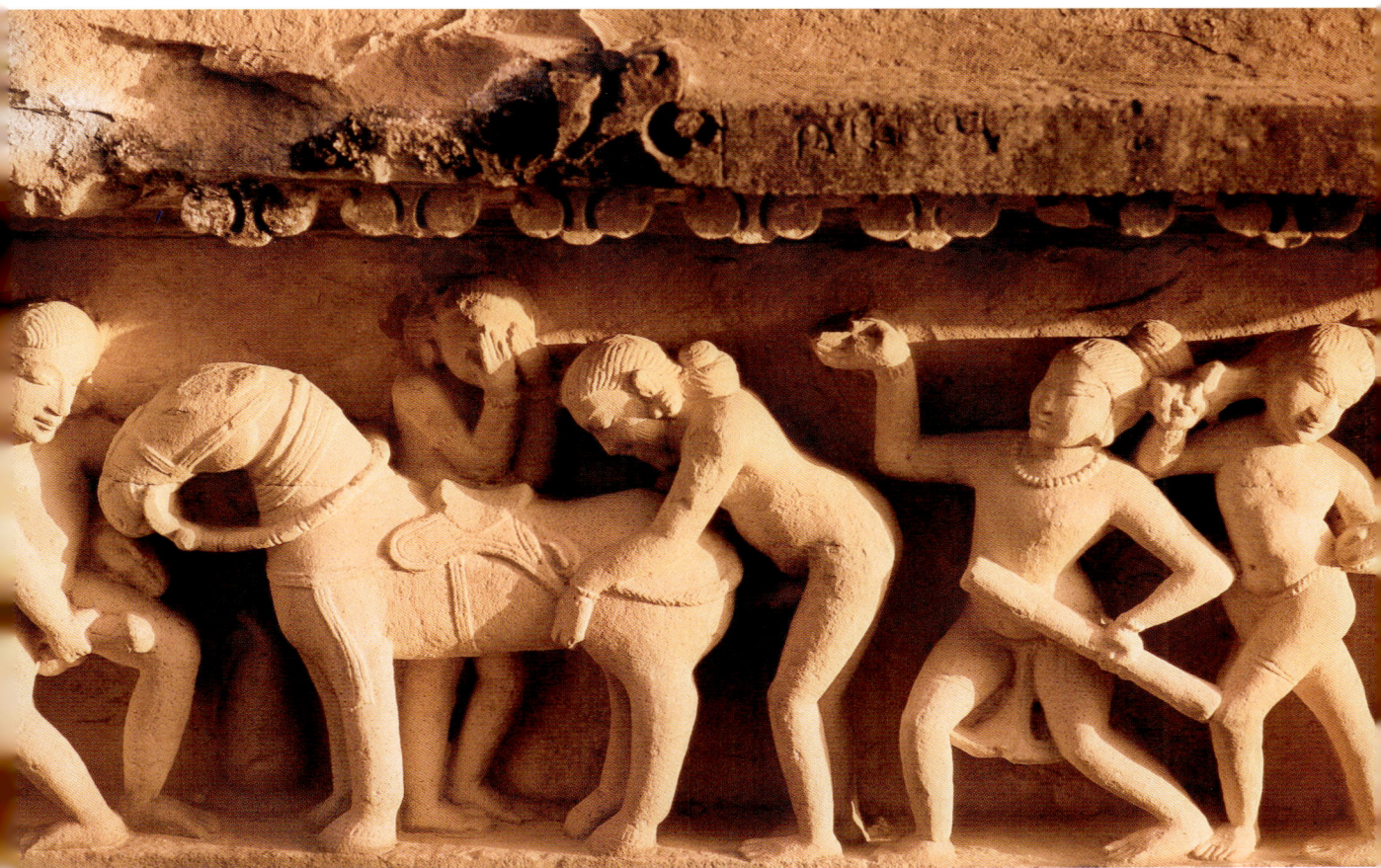

Given the extent of erotic mythologies that abound in world literature, there is little doubt that human sexuality was accepted to be the basis of all human existence. This sense of the erotic became all pervasive in religion, art as well as science touching, impacting and shaping attitudes, behaviour, social aspirations, lifestyles, conduct and values.

The entire range of sexual expressions are found on temple walls—heterosexuality, homosexuality, orgies, bestiality. There are no rules here.

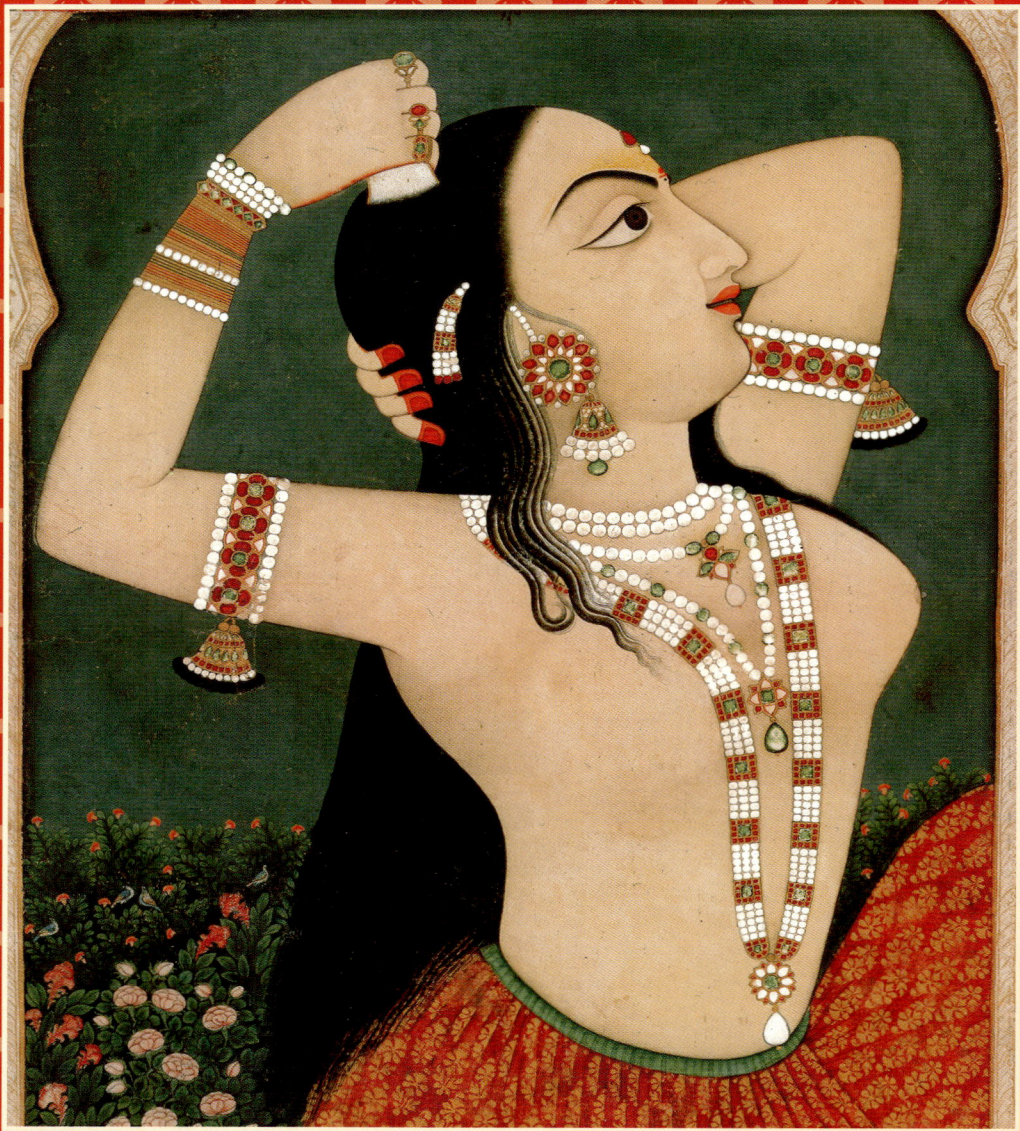

Kama Sutra and Beyond

The term homosexuality translates literally as 'of the same sex', and is a hybrid word from the Greek prefix 'homo' meaning 'same' and the Latin root meaning 'sex'. The term was coined in 1869 by Karl Maria Kertbeny in an anonymous pamphlet advocating the repeal of Prussia's laws on sodomy. It was listed in 1886 in Richard von Krafft-Ebing's detailed study called *Psychopathia Sexualis* dealing with deviant sexual practices. Today the word is used to describe sexual behaviour beween people of the same sex and often causing confusion and controversy.

Several studies, especially *Sexual Behaviour in the Human Male* (1948) and *Sexual Behaviour in the Human Female* (1953), both by Dr Alfred C Kinsey, famously concluded that most people had at least some attraction to either sex, although usually preferring one sex, whereby only a small minority (5-10%) were considered to be fully heterosexual or homosexual. So it would appear that sexual activity with a person of the same sex, in and of itself, does not necessarily demonstrate homosexual orientation. Not all who are attracted or have sexual relationships with members of the same sex identify themselves as homosexual or even bisexual. Some people frequently have sex with members of the same sex yet still see themselves as heterosexual. This is the modern day construct and interpretation on homoeroticism. But ancient cultures and civilizations, not just Indian, regarded sexual identities such as 'homosexuality', 'heterosexuality' or 'bisexuality' as mere social constructions that had to be recognized and accepted without much ado or analysis. Vedic India especially considered all these as natural gender variations and not a social disorder or vice.

In India it is almost impossible to separate eroticism from the fabric of religion, all aspects of human existence being woven into the weft and warp of a way of life that has come to be known as Hinduism. While the task of trying to reconcile preconceived ideas about sexuality and religion may not be an easy one for Western cultures, in India, it was seamless.

In Indian mythology the catchword is *kama* or desire, seen as the first seed that made the very act of creation possible. The governing principle behind *kama* is that of a primal motivator, the cause behind every longing. And this longing can take any shape, size or form. The word *kama* is thus about all types of desire and is defined as the mental inclination toward the pleasures of the senses—touch, sight, taste, and smell. Ancient India had an open attitude towards sexuality without hypocrisy, duplicity or inhibition. Instead of being burdened by guilt, shame and self-consciousness, people were encouraged to study and explore their sexuality and develop the art of loving through education and practice. Satisfaction in every sphere of life was considered the characteristic of civilized society and to this end

Facing page: Sexuality is openly celebrated—without hypocrisy, shame or self-consciousness. Every individual is encouraged to develop the art of loving through practice and education.

० रनाई हुंरमरदंगतालडफबाजै बाजैजंत्रनादसरजै
(३२१) गुणगंधरपत्रकारिखनंगी संगीतकलाकोकरसं
गी गावैनादचृसमुधनकवै मानौ इंद्रसभासुरसवे ॥३४॥ वा
निफिरडलहनीउहल बांधेमोरसेहराफलह उठतफवर

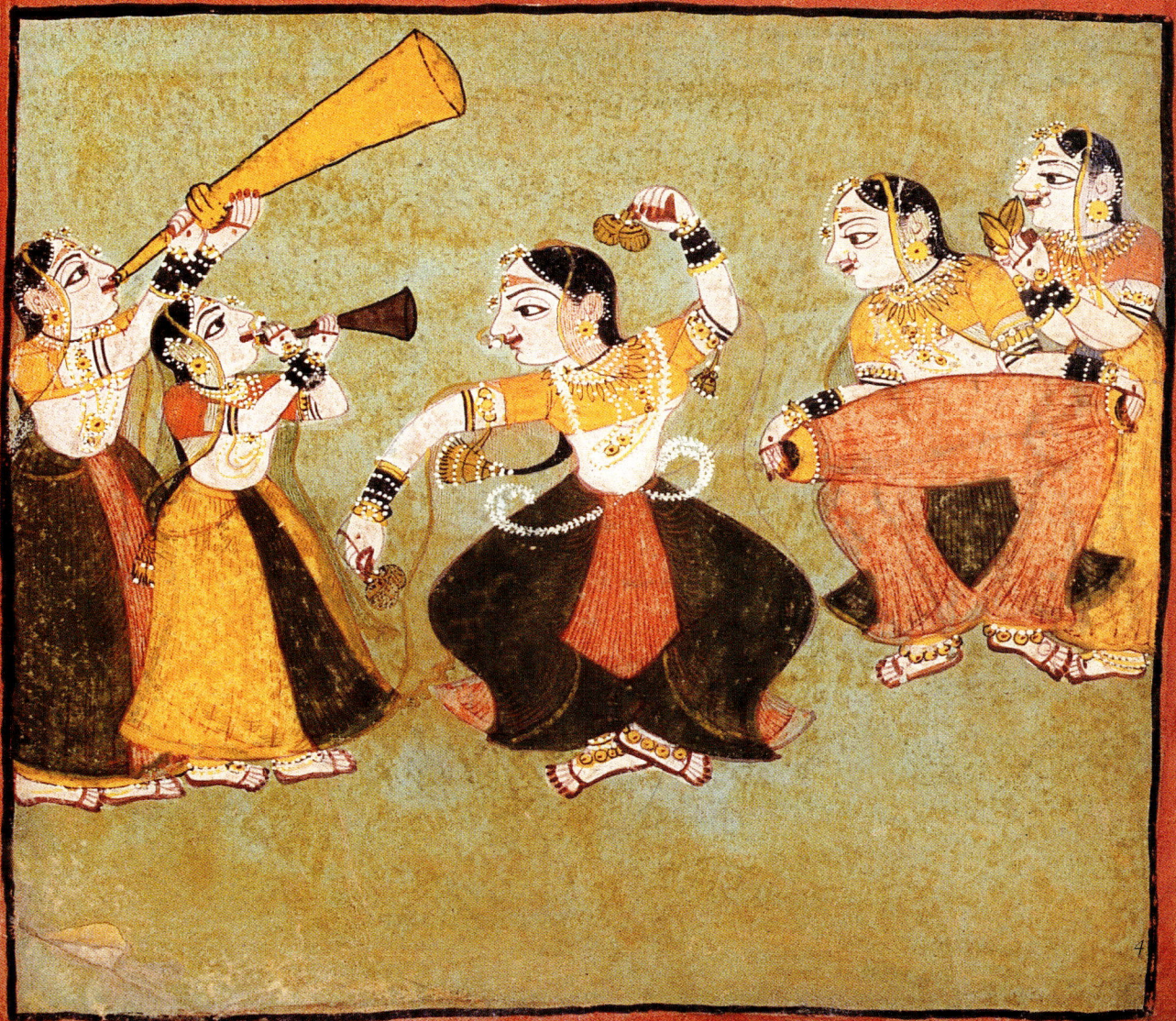

every aspect of life was included. *Kama* would, 'find its finality in itself', being an intrinsic emotion that would find expression for its own gratification.

Between the 2nd and 4th centuries AD, a celibate Brahman monk called Vatsyayana extracted from several older works, a single comprehensive shorter anthology that would cater to society at large. Although widely viewed today as an erotic manual that merely describes impossible, often contorted sexual positions and techniques of intercourse, the *Kama Sutra* provides an alternate window to ancient Hindu heritage. It was not a religious text but a Vedic analysis of the science of human sexuality and gender, similar to other works that analyse different aspects of material science such as the *Dharma Shastra, Artha Shastra, Ayurveda, Dhanurveda,* among others. These texts take such little note of homosexuality that we are led to conclude that Vedic society neither condemned nor felt threatened by its practice. Taking its cue from these earlier texts, the *raison d'être* of the *Kama Sutra* was the acquisition of knowledge, the need for sexual compatibility and the documentation of all aspects of sexuality as well as its variables. There were just no laws that specifically forbade sexual acts between people of the third sex. This viewpoint is further verified by the open discussion of homosexuality within the *Kama Shastra,* and the homosexual acts vividly portrayed

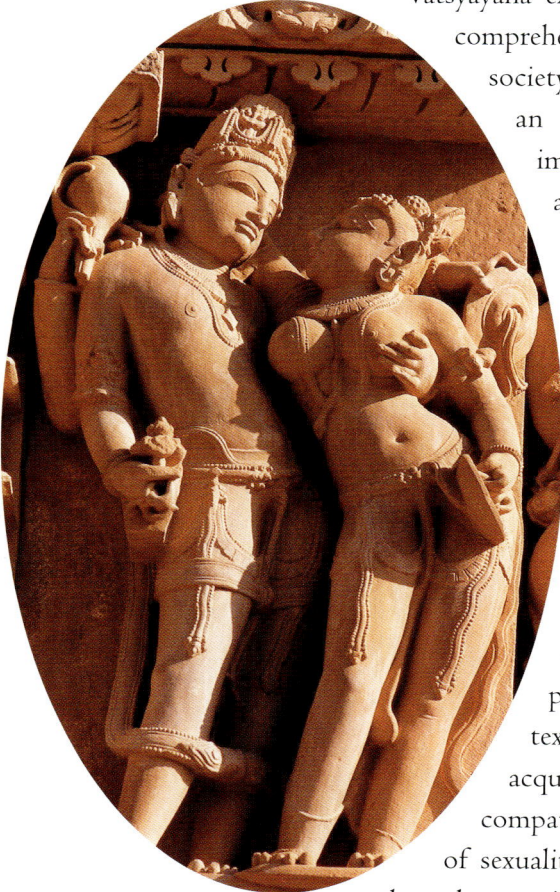

Facing page: The raison d'être *of the* Kama Sutra *was the acquisition of knowledge, and the documentation of all aspects of sexuality as well as its variables.*

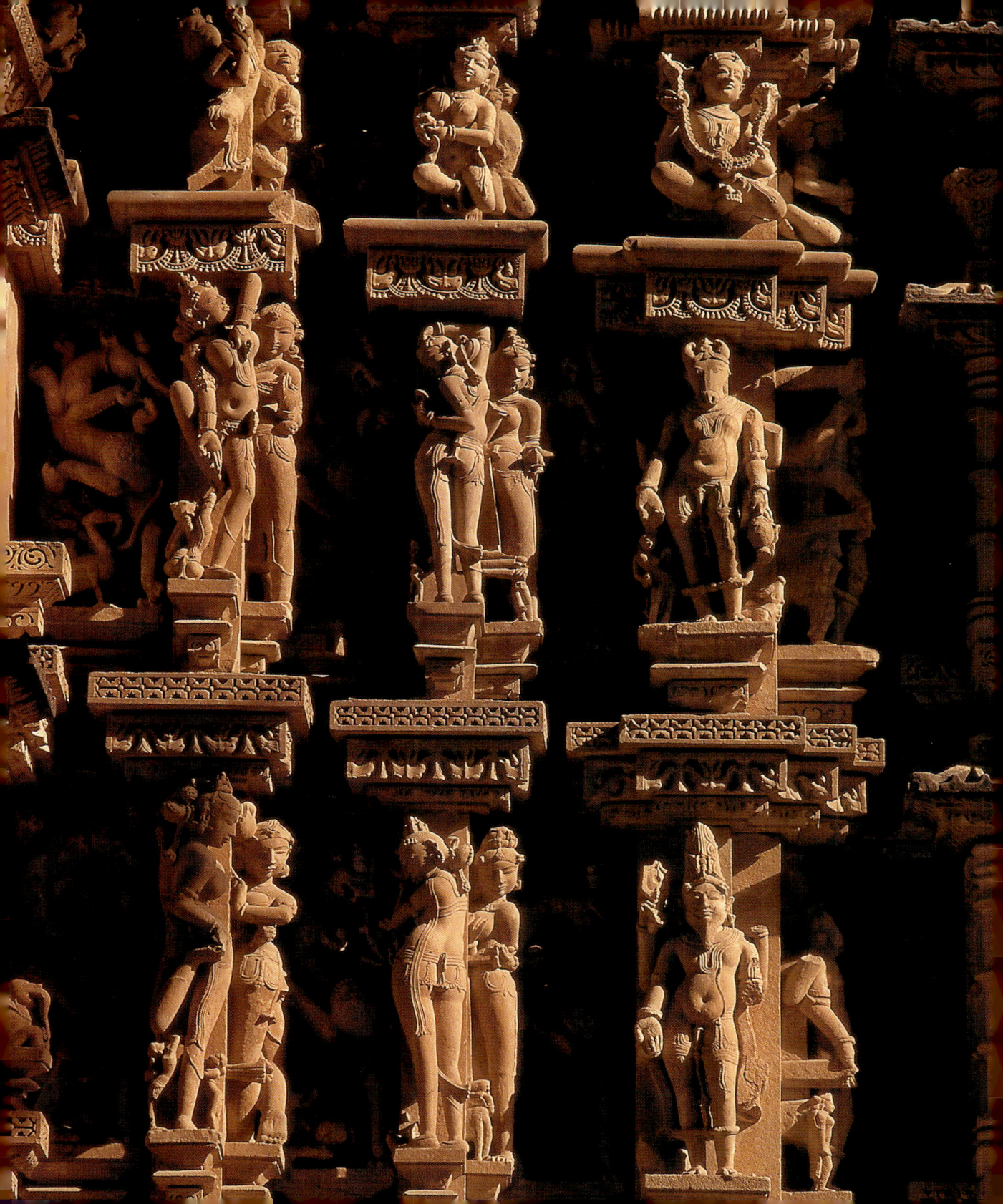

on temple walls in eastern and southern India, especially at Chapri and Khajuraho.

Aesthetics, whether it was art, sculpture, music, poetry or literature, was seen as a refinement and a necessary requirement in the game of love. Understanding that love too was an art and requires outside support without which all modes of expression could very easily become static and repetitive, it was believed that human beings who developed a fine sense of the artistic could use this as a means of communication and self-expression that would enhance relationships. It was believed that being accomplished in the sixty-four arts listed in the *Kama Sutra* guaranteed a person an honorable place in society. More importantly this knowledge would ensure that one would easily win over the object of desire, be it a husband, wife or lover, and provide fulfillment. 'The sixty-four arts should be conceived as the Paths of Creative Energy. They can be likened to the flames of an inner sun, blazing from the solar plexus, burning up all negativity, flames of creativity purify the psyche and bring about an inner transformation,' says Nik Douglas in his book *Sexual Secrets*. Thus besides music, dance, painting, dressing and perfumery it was also advised that, especially women, learnt the art of poetry, massaging, cooking, storytelling, gambling, gardening, mimicry, languages, etiquette, religious rites, household management, physical sports, and martial arts plus many specialized activities related to the culture and time.

The aim of the sixty-four arts was thus not merely to be a good wife, but to be a skilful,

A keenly cultivated sense of aesthetics is seen as a pathway for creative energies to find expression.

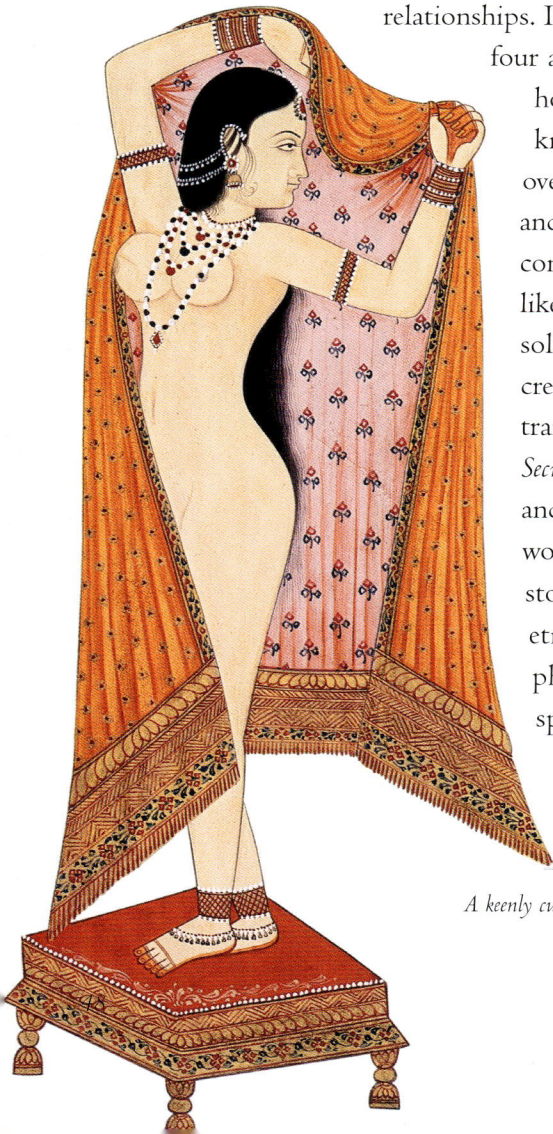

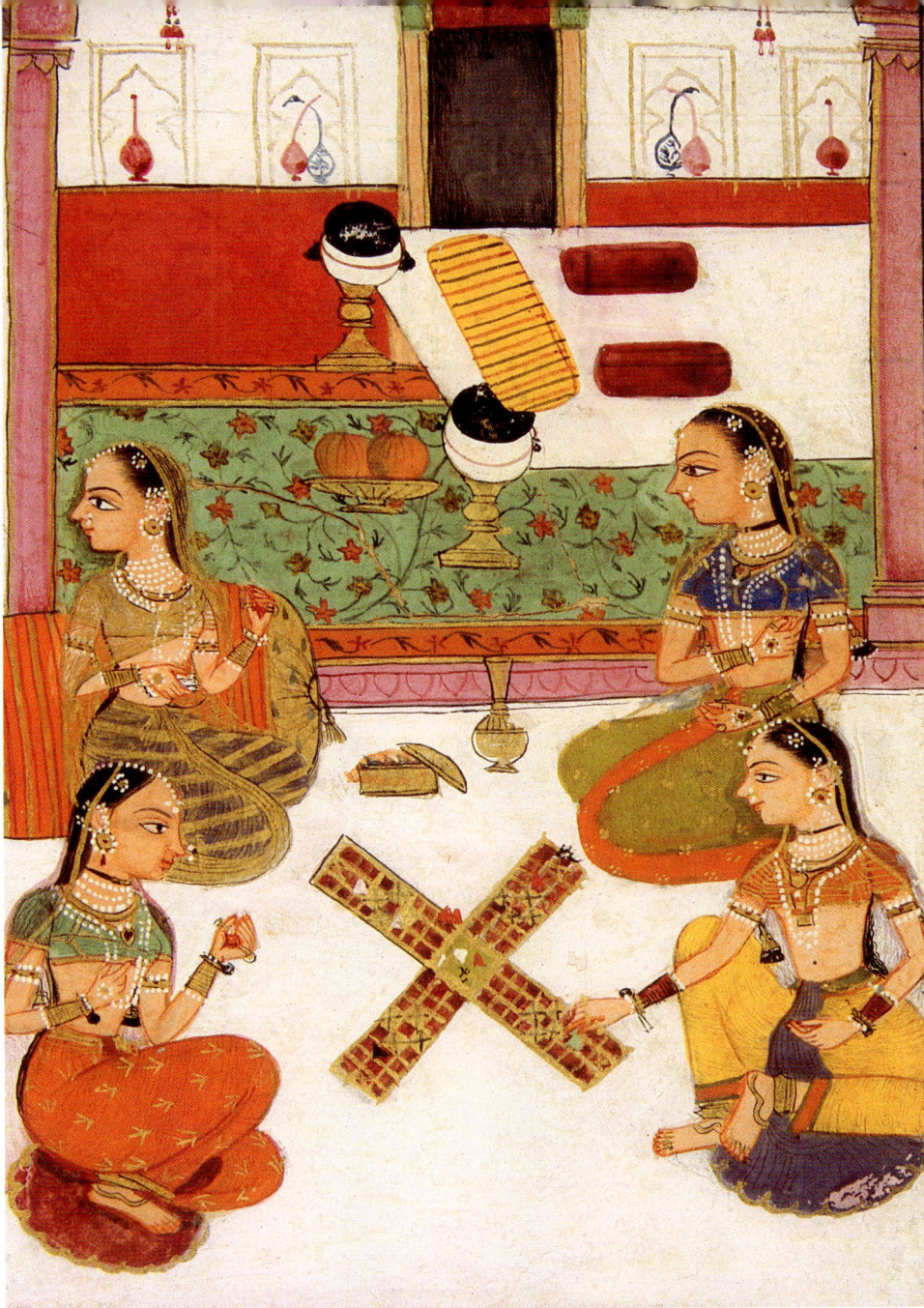

The sixty-four arts were not merely lessons in how to be a good companion, but to be an understanding, intelligent and a refined and sexual human being.

playful, understanding, refined, sexual, beautiful and intelligent woman. The same applied to men too—their need to cultivate an understanding of women and the importance of creating sensual environments and moods for intimacy. The ancient Indians paid great attention to detail of smell, light, music, food, drink and touch before intercourse could begin, all of which gives us a glimpse of the social, cultural and erotic life of a people who were energetic, life affirming, tolerant and surprisingly far ahead of their times.

The seven chapters into which the *Kama Sutra* is divided—General Principles, Sexual Union, Courtship and Marriage, The Wife, Seducing the Wives of Others, Courtesans, and Erotic Lore—provide a valuable insight into the extent of the sexually acceptable, and the depth of the study involved. Ancient India was primarily heterosexual, and marriage was considered to be a logical goal in a respectable and safe relationship between lovers. Monogamy was the norm and based on mutual respect, love, faith and the right to seek mutual sexual fulfillment. The sages of ancient India, however, understood that an absence of sexual happiness in even an otherwise happy marriage would lead to experimentation and result in a multiplicity of partners.

In course of the text, Vatsyayana constantly cites the differing opinions of several scholars, emphasizing at every point that different points of view are possible and that no one opinion can lay any claim to absolute validity. The text also stresses the difference between recommending and permitting, and that variations which are not recommended, may still be permitted, and if not accepted at least recognized. Vatsyayana also cautions that everything that is described in the text does not necessarily have to be performed, 'just as medical texts mention eating dog's flesh for certain illnesses which does not mean this is a recommended edible'. But every type of sex was described because 'there are some people, some occasions and some places where these acts may be performed.' So one should perform or not perform them, bearing the place, time, text, context, and one's own inclinations in mind. But, he continues, 'the mind of the man being fickle, how can it be known what any person will do at any particular time and for what purpose.'

Interestingly no sanctions were pronounced for deviations. So it should come as no surprise that there was no concept of chastity belts in India, no stoning of women for adultery and almost no divorces. In the *Artha Shastra*, for example, minor fines were meted out for homosexual acts committed in public view or within prohibited areas. In fact the maximum penalty that society meted out to deviant behaviour were banal punishments such as ritual baths, donation of cows, chanting of a few hymns and the giving of alms.

As a compendium, the *Kama Sutra* attempts to exhaust all possibilities and to mention every possible type of sexual behaviour. So, in keeping with the social milieu of the time, courtesans *(ganikas)* were respected and accepted as part of social life as were temporary relationships, contractual arrangements, relationships with housemaids, and pleasure houses run by women trained in the art and craft of love. Sex with animals, manual sex between women, the making and use of dildos and penis sheaths, piercing of sex organs, different types of group sex, imitation of animal sex, and what are today called sadomasochistic practices such as biting, scratching, and beating, even to the point of killing the partner (the last of these is definitively condemned), are all described. Neither are other aspects of sexuality ignored—same-sex love is accepted and acknowledged as are all gender perspectives: men, women, homosexuals, lesbians, prostitutes, and eunuchs or persons of the 'third nature'.

THE THIRD SEX

What does the 'third nature' stand for? What category of people does it constitute? Do these divisions exist in present-day society?

The very fact that these classifications were noted, studied and penned down with great care in the *Kama Shastra* and other sociological and moral texts of Vedic India demonstrates the acceptance of an intermediary gender construct apart from the accepted norm of men and women. Gender, as seen in the Introduction was divided into *pums-prakrti* (the nature of men), *striya-prakrti* (the nature of women) and *tritiya-prakrti* (the third nature). These three divisions were based not only on physical characteristics but rather on an assessment of the entire human being that included the physical, psychological, emotional and social interaction which in this case took into account their ability to procreate. A forerunner to the Kinsey Reports (some 1700 years ahead of time), the 8th and 9th chapters of the *Kama Sutra* describes the third sex as a natural gradation of the male and female natures to the point where they can no longer be categorized as male or female in the traditional sense of the word.

Gays

This third category was further classified into *napumsakas* and *svairinis*. The exact definition of the word '*napumsaka*' has been widely debated, but is generally accepted to mean a person who is neither man nor woman. The book describes five different types of people who can be *napumsakas*: (1) children (2) the elderly (3) neuters (4) the celibate, and (5) the third sex. By Vedic definition, they were all considered to be sexually neutral, belonging to a distinct social category, and who did not engage in sexual reproduction.

The word '*napumsaka*' can thus refer to any non-reproductive member of society, who is usually described as male but is actually a member of the third sex. These men in turn are divided into two types—*strirupini* and *purusharupini*—those who choose who take the *rupa* or appearance of a *stri* or woman: 'those with a feminine appearance show it by their dress, speech, laughter, behaviour, gentleness, lack of courage, silliness, patience, and modesty.' The other category comprises those who were like *purushas* or masculine in appearance and have moustaches and beards. Men who dress up as females were then as today known as transvestites. Feminine gay males were often professionally employed by aristocratic women and commonly served within the royal palace. They were proficient in the arts, entertainment and most notably dancing. Masculine gay males are next described as 'those who like

Facing page: Lesbian women in ancient India were known as 'independent women'— ones who refused to marry, earned their own living and managed their own affairs.

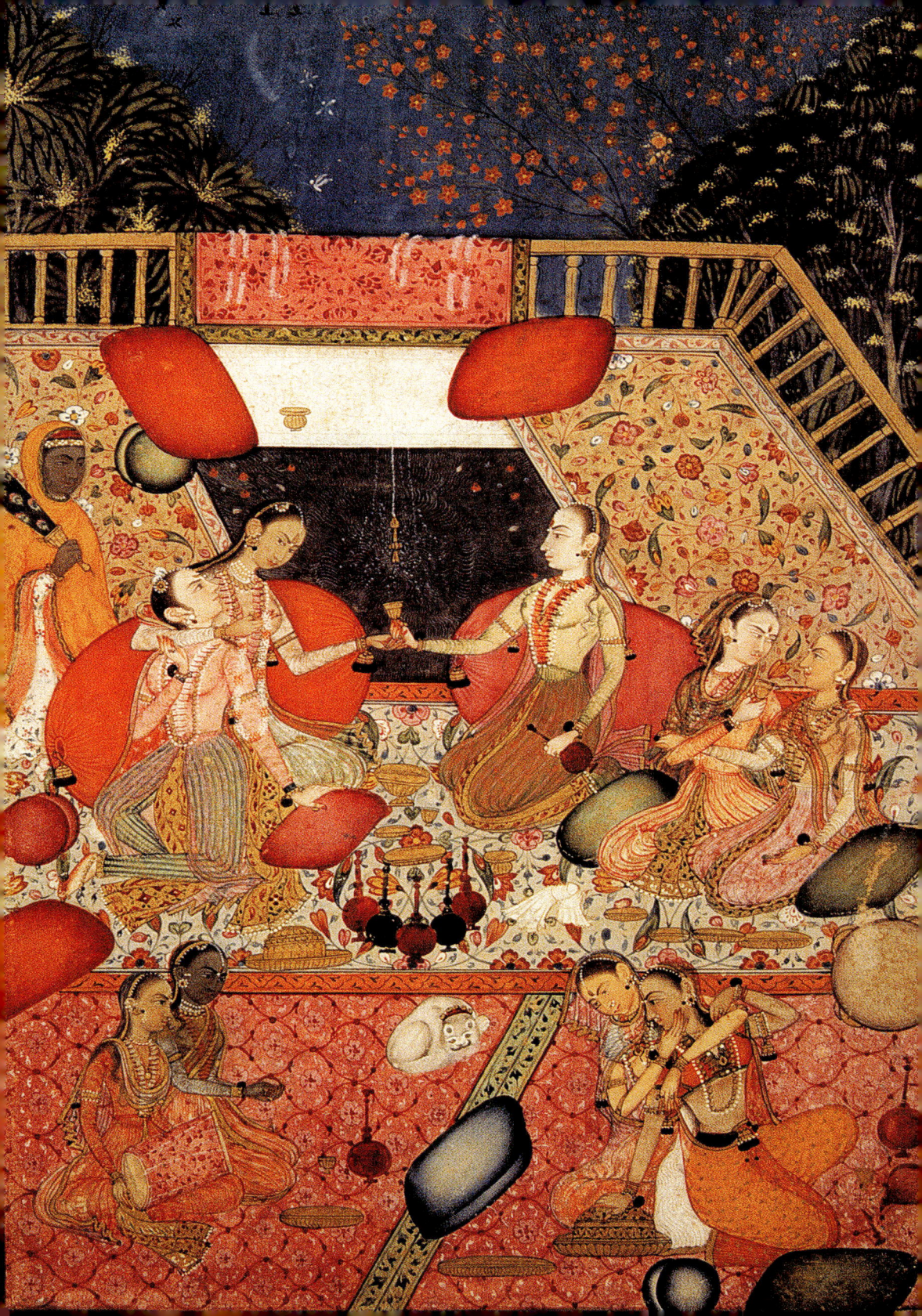

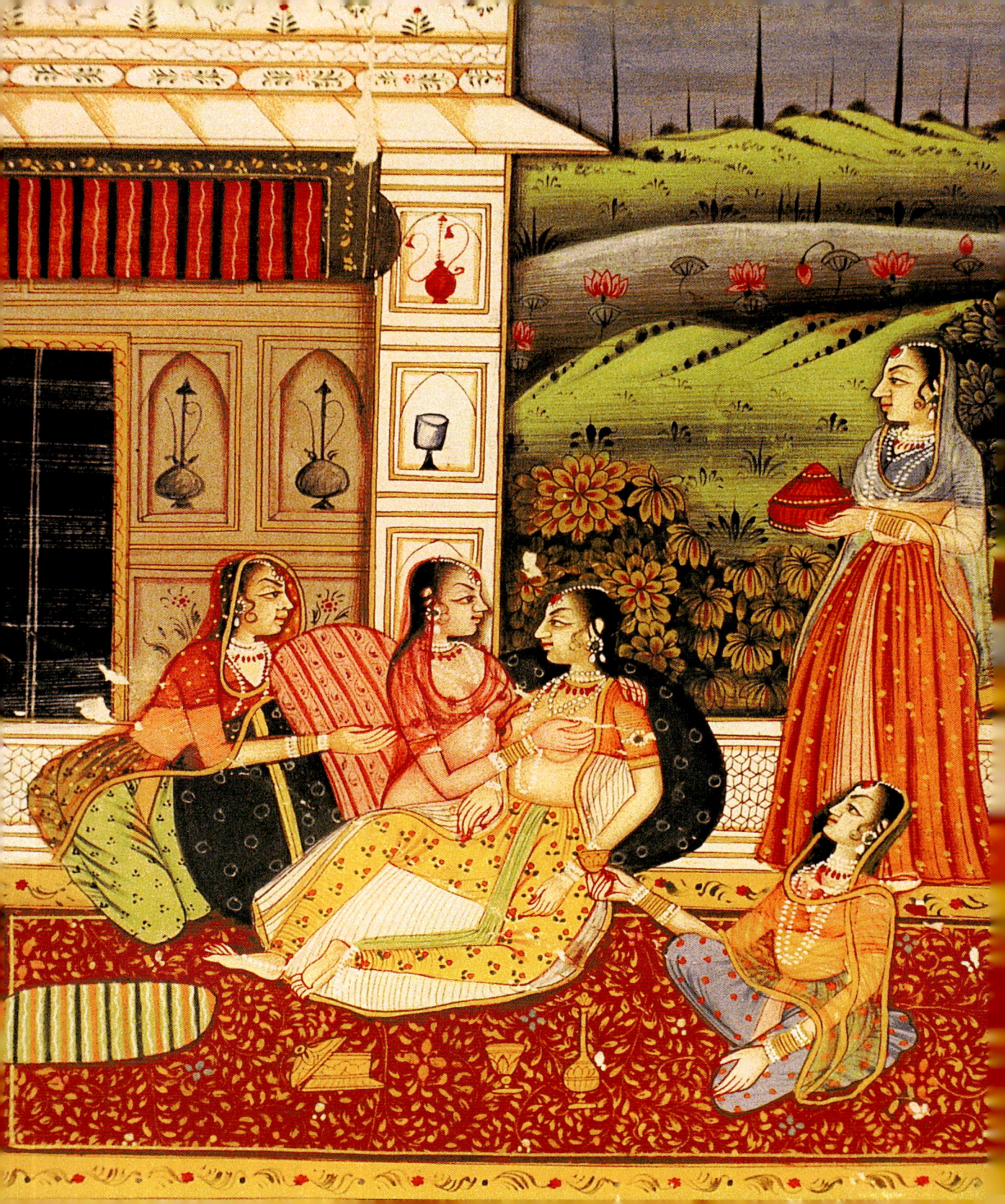

men but dissimulate the fact, maintain a manly appearance, and earn their living as barbers or masseurs.' The masculine gay male is therefore not easily recognizable and often blends in, living either independently or within marriage to another man. While effeminate gay men are described as those with smooth skin, using make-up and oftentimes sporting shiny earrings; the more masculine gays would keep bodily hair, grow moustaches or small beards and maintain a muscular physique.

Another Sanskrit word that appears rather early in literature and is used to describe gay men is *kliba*. In the *Atharva Veda* hymns that were compiled between the 7th and 8th century BC, there is mention of *kliba*s or long-haired men who wore women's head ornaments. In verse of the same Veda, the *kliba*s cast spells to make men impotent. Elsewhere there is reference to a charm that protects pregnant women from demons, and in which the 'wild dance of the long-haired men' is described. Other words that were used to describe gays were *sanda, panda* and *hijra*, all of which have a wide range of meanings— those who were sterile, impotent, castrated, transvestites, men who had oral sex with other men, ones who had anal sex, men with mutilated or defective sexual organs, as well as hermaphrodites.

Lesbians

In the *Kama Sutra*, lesbians are described as women who exhibit aggressive behaviour like men *(purushayita)*. The Sanskrit word for lesbian is *svairini* though the word literally means a liberated woman who refuses to marry, earns and manages her own finances and lives either alone or in marriage with another woman. According to the societal norms of the time, lesbians were more likely to marry and raise children than their male counterparts and were thus readily accommodated both within the third-gender community and ordinary society. In her book *Sakhiyani*, Gita Thadani addresses the difficulty inherent in using the term 'lesbian' to describe ancient female-to female eroticism. She says, '...lesbian is a post-industrial/Western term,

Facing page: The svairini *woman was known for her independence, had no sexual barriers and made love with her own kind.*

a social construction'. Clearly, the absence of such definition does not prevent lesbianism from existing. *Svairini* also known as *narisandha, sandha,* or *sandhi* are thus independent women who frequent their own kind or others, and have relationships in their own homes or in other houses. 'A woman known for her independence, with no sexual bars, and acting as she wishes, is called *svairini*. She makes love with her own kind. She strokes her partner at the point of union, which she kisses. Once she has won the girl's trust, the *svairini* practises the acts mentioned above, pitilessly, ill-treating the girl's pubis.'

The *Kama Sutra* does indeed discuss 'Female-female sexual activity' but less overtly and more as a 'situational behaviour found among women in sexually segregated environments (such as the women's quarters), rather than as an essential characteristic or pathology of certain individuals'. According to Vatsyayana, there is a great deal of lesbian activity within harems. Here, due to the absence of men, women use dildos, as well as bulbs, roots, or fruits that have the form of the male organ, and statues of men that have distinct sexual characteristics. Not that lesbian activity in the modern sense did not exist—according to the *Manusmriti,* 'a woman who corrupts a virgin will be punished by having two of her fingers cut off, a hint of what Manu thinks lesbians do in bed.' The *Kama Sutra* discusses female virile activities, where women sodomize men, seduce and penetrate another woman with a dildo. Some of the descriptions of 'virile copulation' (*purushopasriptani*) are quite graphic: 'churning, the rod, the devastator, the cruel, the thunderbolt, the wild boar's thrust, and the bull's blow' are among the more eye-catching ones. 'Churning' involved lowering the one to be penetrated onto a protruding object spinning on a potter's wheel. The 'devastator' caused vibrations by shaking the 'rod' violently while penetrating the other woman with it. 'Normal copulation' between the two women involved the use of a 'rectilinear object'. The penetrator was called *svairini. Svairini*s were also possibly oral sex partners and prostitutes. Buccal coition was said to be practised with corrupt women (*kulata*), lesbians (*svairini*), servants (*paricharika*), women who carry burdens (*sanvahika*). The various kinds of prostitutes are: the water carrier (*kumbhad-visi*), the servant (*paricharika*), the corrupt woman (*kulata*), the lesbian (*svairini*), the dancer (*nati*), the worker (*shilparika*), the divorcee or widow

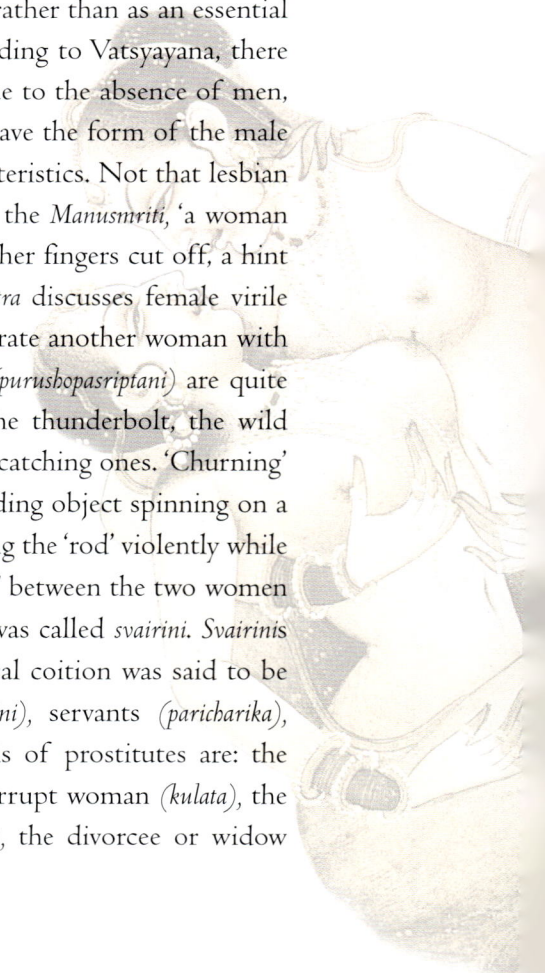

(*prakashavinashta*), the harlot who lives on her own charms (*rupajiva*), and the courtesan (*ganika*). In the *Jayamangala,* an important 12th-century commentary on the *Kama Sutra,* according to Yashodhara, such behaviour among women was not forbidden.

In fact, considerable evidence suggests that female homoerotic relationships were commonplace in the harem (*zenana*). Although the concept of a harem did not exist in Vedic India and was a latter-day addition, the *zenana* became a homosocial institution where women were usually secluded from all men except their husbands and sons. The *Kama Sutra* contains an early description of such eroticism within harems: 'As a protective measure, nobody may enter the inner apartments. There is only one husband, while the wives, who are often several, remain unsatisfied. This is why, in practice, they have to obtain satisfaction among themselves. The nurse's daughter, female companions, and slaves, dressed as men, take the men's place and use carrots, fruits, and other objects to satisfy their desire'. In some harems, the art of rubbing clitoris against clitoris is taught and every girl becomes well versed in the Sapphic sciences. 'To solace her in long hours of desire for the male, nearly every concubine had her own private companion with whom she practices all the Sapphic pleasures.'

In a rather amusing account written by a 16th-century Venetian envoy about Ottoman harems, vegetables such as cucumbers were banned from use for erotic enjoyment: 'It is not lawful for anyone to bring aught in unto them [the women of the harem] with which they may commit deeds of beastly uncleanliness; so that if they have a will to eat Cucumbers, they are sent in unto them sliced to deprive them of the means of playing the wantons.' While some controversy exists over this custom in Ottoman harems, it appears from the *Kama Sutra* that bans such as these were not imposed in India where the absence of men is the most common excuse deployed as the reason for female homoeroticism in a gender-segregated environment. So, according to Vatsyayana, citizens dressed as women are sometimes introduced into the harem with the maidservants. They are assisted in their comings and goings by the nurses or the other harem women who hoped to benefit financially. 'The maidservants explain to them that entry is easy and the guards are not there all the time. If the way is not easy, men should renounce the task, since the matter is risky.' (*Kama Sutra* 5.6.6-9). It was thus possible for women deprived of men to obtain male sex partners. In some areas harems were not closely guarded, and men could enter. In others, entry was easily obtained on days of the full moon and the festival of lights, or 'by way of the vaults' (5.6.26). 'In Vindarbha, the queens slept with all the princes except their own sons' (5.6.32). Though Vatsyayana warns the man of the dangers of entering a harem and generally advises against such behaviour, he acknowledges that a man who was in the 'grip of violent passion' would find entry anyway, even go 'every day' if invited. (5.6.10-20).

Besides, the *Kama Sutra* also advises wives on how to interact and behave with their husband's other wives. The good wife was to sleep next to the elder women of the household when her husband was absent and to develop intimate relationships with them. In the harems some kings slept with wives in turn, one per night; others slept mostly with favorites; still others, who were more considerate to their wives, slept with all or many of them at one time (5.6). As there was only one man and many women in such a situation, female homoeroticism could be incorporated. In the *Kama Sutra*, group sex involving one man and several women is compared to a 'bull' with a 'herd of cows *(goyuthi)*.

BISEXUALITY

Besides men who had sexual relationships with one another, women within and outside harems too conducted affairs with their own sex. The *Kama Sutra* as well as other treatises on sexuality acknowledges the presence of another gender group, who are today known as bisexuals. However, in Vedic times, bisexuality was considered to be more of a variation for heterosexual men and women who were so inclined, and not as a category of the third sex. Since categorization was based on the ability or inability to have children, and as several bisexuals did procreate, they were not

Facing page: The Kama Sutra *categorizes people who are bisexual as those who have an excessive desire to have intercourse.*

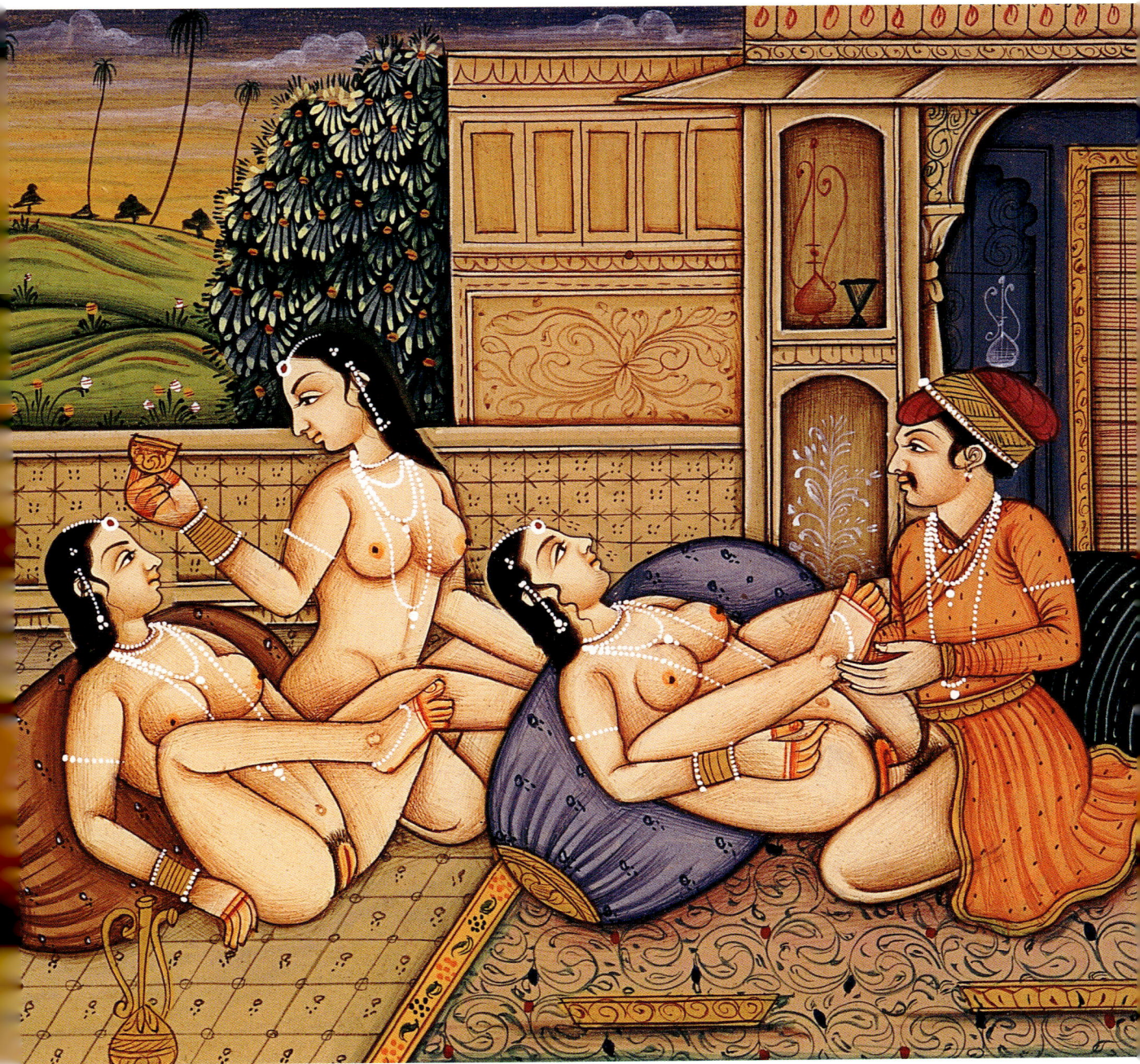

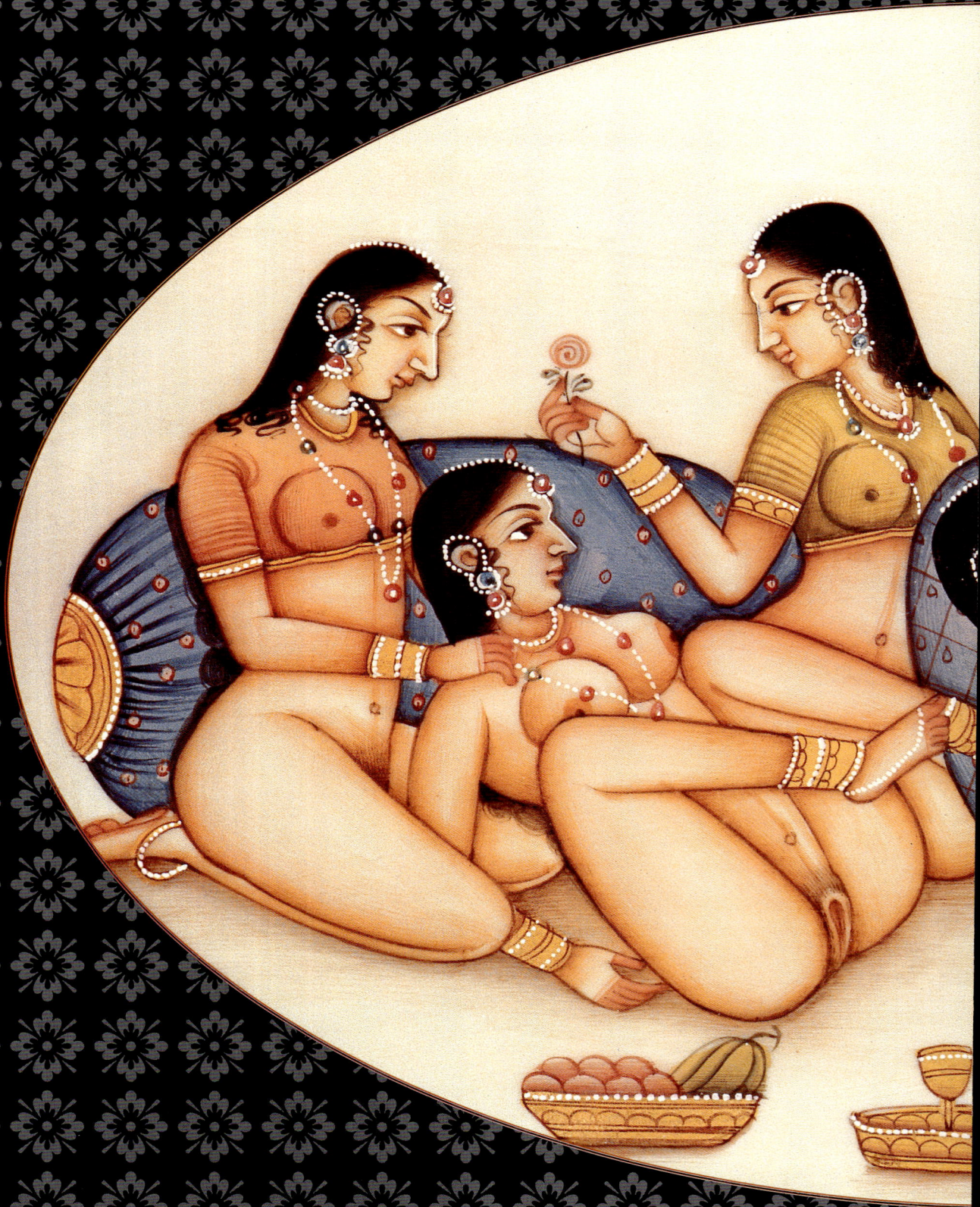

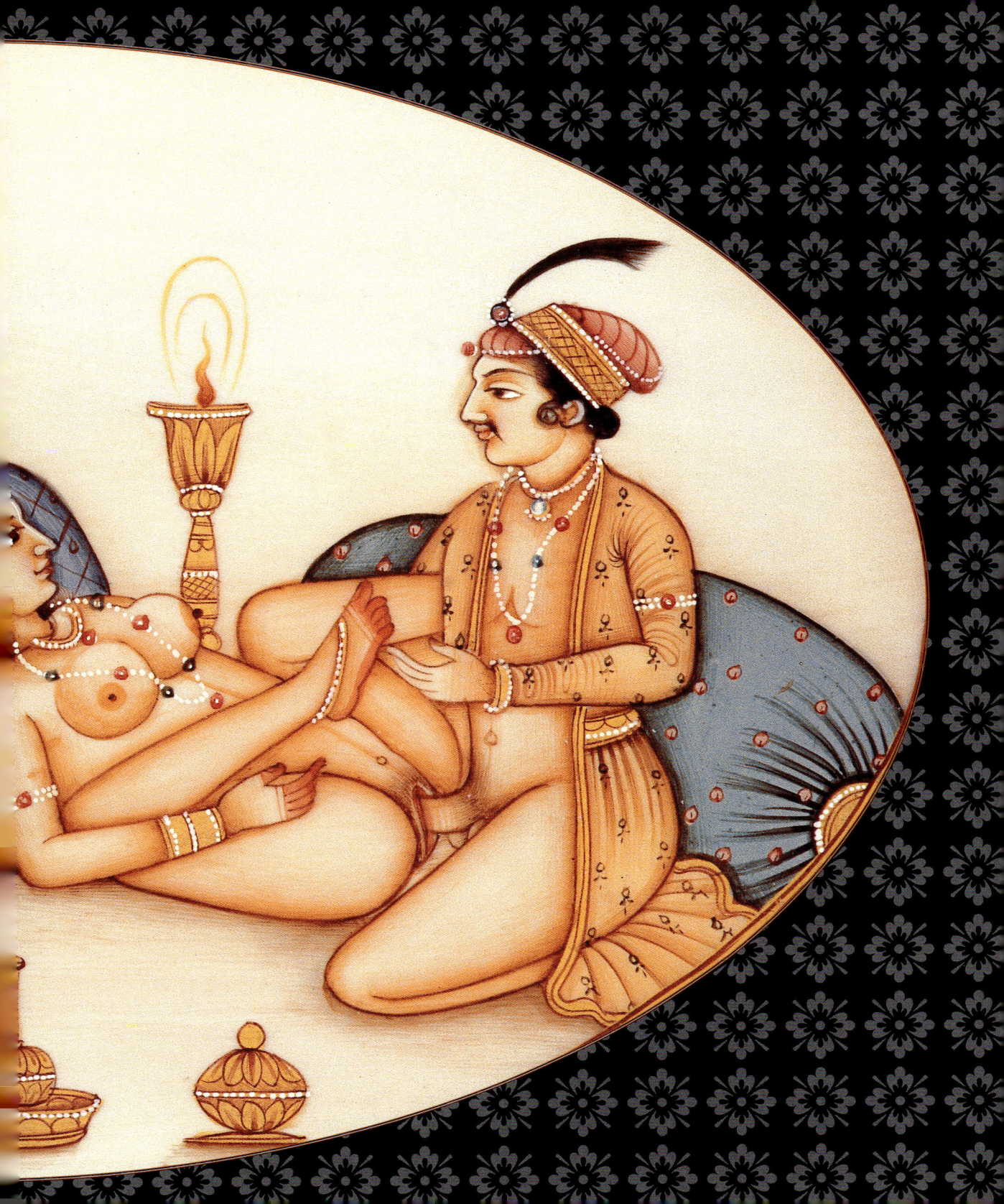

considered to be *napumsakas* or sexually neutral people. The Sanskrit word for bisexuals is *kami* which means one who is excessively desirous of making love. The *Kama Shastra* thus discusses men who visit transvestites or masseurs working as prostitutes, men in the company of lesbians, transvestites within the king's harem, women of the harem satisfying themselves during the king's absence, and male servants who practice homosexuality in their youth but then later become inclined towards women.

As Zia Jaffery says in her book *The Invisibles*, which examines the tale of eunuchs in India, 'there was poetry to the idea of the third sex... for whom, society provided a "welfare system".' Women and men of the third sex were engaged in all means of livelihood including trade, government, entertainment, as courtesans or prostitutes, as masseurs and maidservants, sometimes living as renunciants and following ascetic vows. There wasn't just a place for everyone in Indian society but a purpose as well. So gay men found their vocation as masseurs. Also known for their fierce loyalty and devotion to their masters they worked as house attendants to wealthy merchants or as chamberlains and ministers to government officials. Celibate homosexuals became temple priests. Feminine gay males were proficient in the arts, entertainment and most notably dancing.

SAME-SEX MARRIAGE

The tolerance with which ancient societies accepted what nature had crafted is best demonstrated by the numerous instances of same-sex marriages that were recorded in ancient India—an idea that is causing a great deal of angst to present-day society. 'There are third-sexed citizens, sometimes greatly attached to each other who with complete faith in one another, get married (*parigraha*),' says the *Kama Sutra*. There were eight different types of marriage according to the Vedic system, and the homosexual marriage that occurred between gay males or lesbians was classified under the Gandharva or celestial variety. The Gandharva marriage is defined as a

---

Preceding pages 60-61: Ancient societies accepted a wide range of sexual practices.

union of love and co-habitation, recognized under common law, but without the need of parental consent or religious sanction. Though Brahmins were prohibited from having this type of marriage, other communities often took part in such ceremonies. The *Jayamangala* states: 'Citizens with this kind of [homosexual] inclination, who renounce women and can do without them willingly because they love each other, get married together, bound by a deep and trusting friendship.' The argument in favour of the acceptance and tolerance of Gandharva weddings was that since the objective of all good relationships is love, this kind of wedding too was respected, even though conducted under unfavourable circumstances, because it fulfilled the purpose. Another reason was that it brought happiness, caused less trouble in its performance than the other types of weddings and most importantly was contracted as a result of love between two consenting people.

LATTER-DAY TEXTS

As the sage Vatsyayana himself says, the *Kama Sutra* was not the first text on erotology, rather a compendium of much earlier works. But compiled as it was sometime during the 3rd century AD, it bridges the gap between the periods that we term as ancient and medieval. The *Kama Sutra* has become the definitive book on Indian eroticism but several latter-day works, such as the 12th-century *Jayamangala* by Yashodhara, carry forward the scholarly practice of accretive composition. Between the 10th and 18th centuries, several texts similar to the *Kama Sutra* were written, most of them by noblemen and kings, who refined the art of courtship and lovemaking while adding their own experiences and interpretations. There were reasons why the middle ages saw an explosion of erotic texts after a hiatus of almost 800 years. For one, the curiosity and interest in sexuality continued unabated. Having already established a tradition of being a sensuous society, the attempt was to keep alive the tradition of knowing what to do, as well as the proper manner and techniques to do it. These texts like Pandit Kokkaka's *Kokashastra*, Kalyanamalla's *Ananga Ranga*, carried forward this knowledge through the medieval period both in Sanskrit and other regional languages and like the *Kama Sutra*, based their studies on the principle of physical gratification, and the premise that pleasure was the ultimate goal even in a patriarchal social structure.

One hitherto unpublished text known as the *Manmata Samhita* explains the main divisions of sexuality thus: 'Oh my beloved! Surat is just another name for sex. It has two main divisions and several sub-sections...Intercourse with women (heterosexual sex) is the first kind, the second is anal sex (which could be both heterosexual or homosexual), the third is masturbation (using one's own hands), and the fourth is to use artificial devices like dildos.'

Additional information about other gender-variants appears in several ancient Sanskrit medical treatises such as the *Caraka Samhita* and the *Susruta Samhita*. In the *Caraka Samhita*, gender and sexual variance is attributed to biological causes. Women with varying sexual propensities are also mentioned in the *Srimad Bhagavatam*. 'Simply by yawning, the demon Bala created three kinds of women, known as *svairinis*, *kaminis* and *pumscalis*. The *svairinis* like to marry men from their own group, the *kaminis* marry men from any group, and the *pumscalis* change husbands one after another. If a man enters the planet of Atala, these women immediately capture him and induce him to drink an intoxicating beverage made with a drug known as *hataka (cannabis indica)*. This intoxicant endows the man with great sexual prowess, of which the women take advantage for enjoyment. A woman will enchant him with attractive glances, intimate words, smiles of love and then embraces. In this way she induces him to enjoy sex with her to her full satisfaction. Because of his increased sexual power, the man thinks himself stronger than ten thousand elephants and considers himself most perfect.'

Vedic civilization recognized and accepted gay men and women in their society, but within limits. Reading the *Kama Sutra*, may lead one to believe that society in those times was licentious, and that the scriptures exhorted a life of hedonistic pleasure. To the contrary, scriptural law of ancient India imposed penalties on those who transgressed its provisions. While various concessions were granted for different

Facing page: An important factor to be considered is one of tolerance and balance. To eschew a life of mere hedonistic pleasure while still seeking one's pleasures with responsibility is an essential lesson.

segments of the third-sex, there were also penalties for transgression. Then, as now, homosexual promiscuity lead to disease for those involved, adultery, divorces, broken families, and other social problems. For this reason, the *Dharma Shastra* and other Vedic texts strictly enforced the institution of marriage among heterosexual couples for the maintenance of the social order. Amara dasa Wilhelm explains it further in his book called the *Third Gender:* 'From the Vedic perspective sexual restraint was only fully effective when it was voluntary. Laws were used to regulate "vice" by establishing designated areas within the city or town and strictly prohibiting it elsewhere, such as in the Brahmin or temple districts. Responsible family life and celibacy were publicly encouraged and promoted by the government, but at the same time other forms of sexual behaviour were acknowledged and accommodated accordingly. Anyone familiar with Vedic literature will be well aware that these activities were allotted a limited space within its culture.'

The important factor that emerges from the *Kama Sutra* is the fact of tolerance. While society was largely heterosexual and monogamy was the norm, even so, the acceptance of variations in gender and relationships, the forbearance shown towards men who became women in their desire for other men, women who opted to be independent and seek their own professions and pleasure, men and women who sought and found oral and anal sex and whatever else took their fancy, only confirms the modernity and maturity of ancient India.

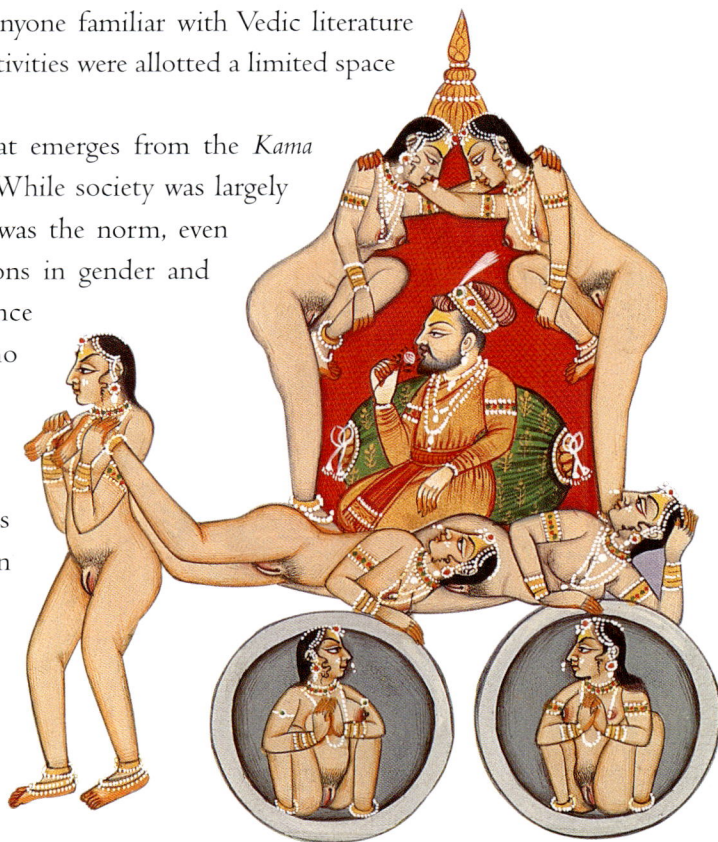

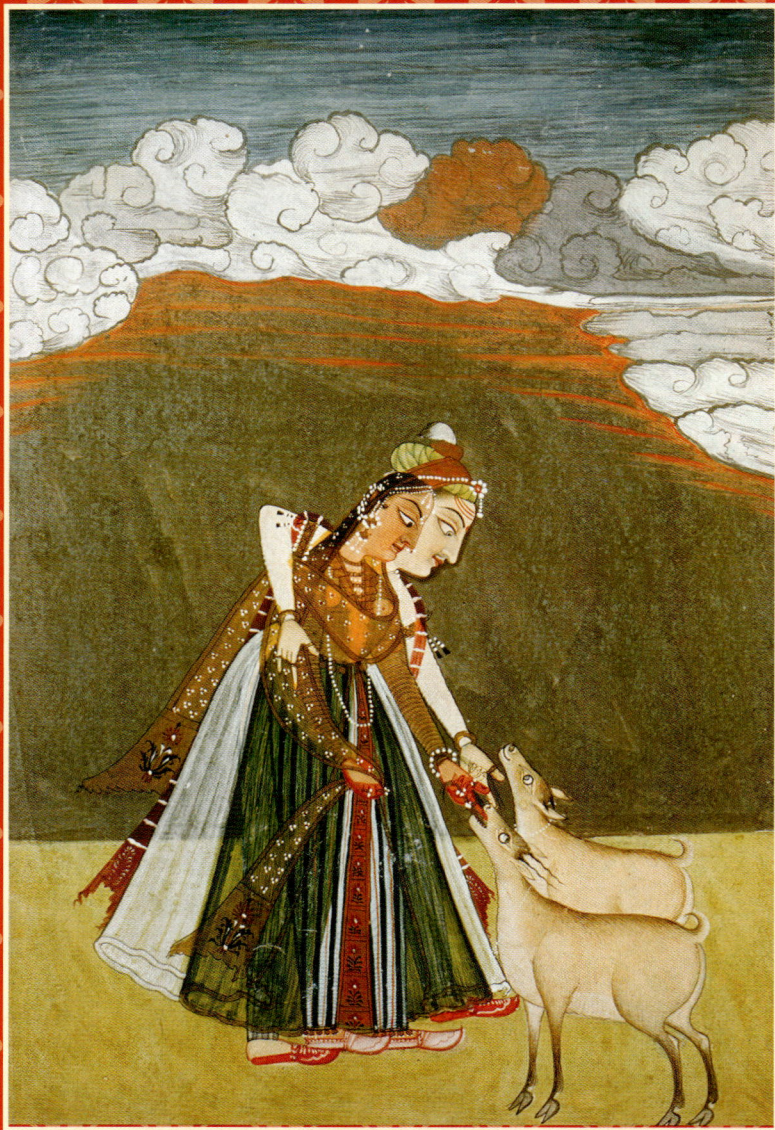

Erotic overtures

The erotic dance between human beings commences at first sight. The frisson of excitement when eye contact is made holding out the promise of an enticing sexual destiny, the senses that come alive with every sight, sound, touch and nuance of the beloved, the sensation in the pit of the stomach, the unspoken word, all carry a message of sensuality that is far more powerful than the physicality of sex.

The emotional comfort that one draws from cuddling a lover, the sense of being wanted and loved, the care that stems from attentiveness are much the same in all human beings whether heterosexual or homosexual. 'Because they belong to the same species, man and woman seek the same pleasure in sexual relations. This is why desire must first be stimulated by preliminary attentions,' says the sage Vatsyayana emphasizing the importance of foreplay so as to master the game of flirting and the nuances of preliminary pleasures. In all cultures first impressions have a habit of becoming lasting impressions, so correct behaviour, a pleasant demeanour, attention to dressing and personal hygiene and a genuine interest in the other person, are prerequisites not merely to engage in the game of seduction but also to build a relationship that endures. The beginning of courtship enhances passion, which leads to foreplay.

What constitutes primary attention? What has made foreplay so important especially now where it occupies premium shelf space and prime time slots as magazines and talk shows promote foreplay as being as important, if not more relevant and satisfying than actual intercourse? The focus is on attentiveness, the feeling of being wanted and relevant; that a person cares enough to spend time to understand, explore and address your needs. Foreplay heightens the sense of sensuousness, slowly building up to a crescendo that will culminate in the actual act of intercourse. Without this sense of erotic connectedness, the physicality of sex remains empty and unsatisfying. It provides an opportunity to express genuine interest in and understand what your partner likes and needs, to be fully stimulated. Foreplay is not the purview of only heterosexuals or young people; even older couples, especially, those who have been in long-term relationships need the extra stimuli to get fully aroused and derive maximum pleasure. The most erogenous zone in the human body is of course the mind where desire first makes its appearance. Ancient civilizations that understood the genesis of desire evolved elaborate mythologies around its birth; for example, the Indian equivalent of Cupid, Kama, is also known as Manasija or the one born of the mind! Every stimulus begins in the mind, as does the arousal of all the senses. So rather than being seen only as physical, desire and arousal are more about

---

Facing page: Foreplay heightens sensuousness building up to the crescendo of actual intercourse.

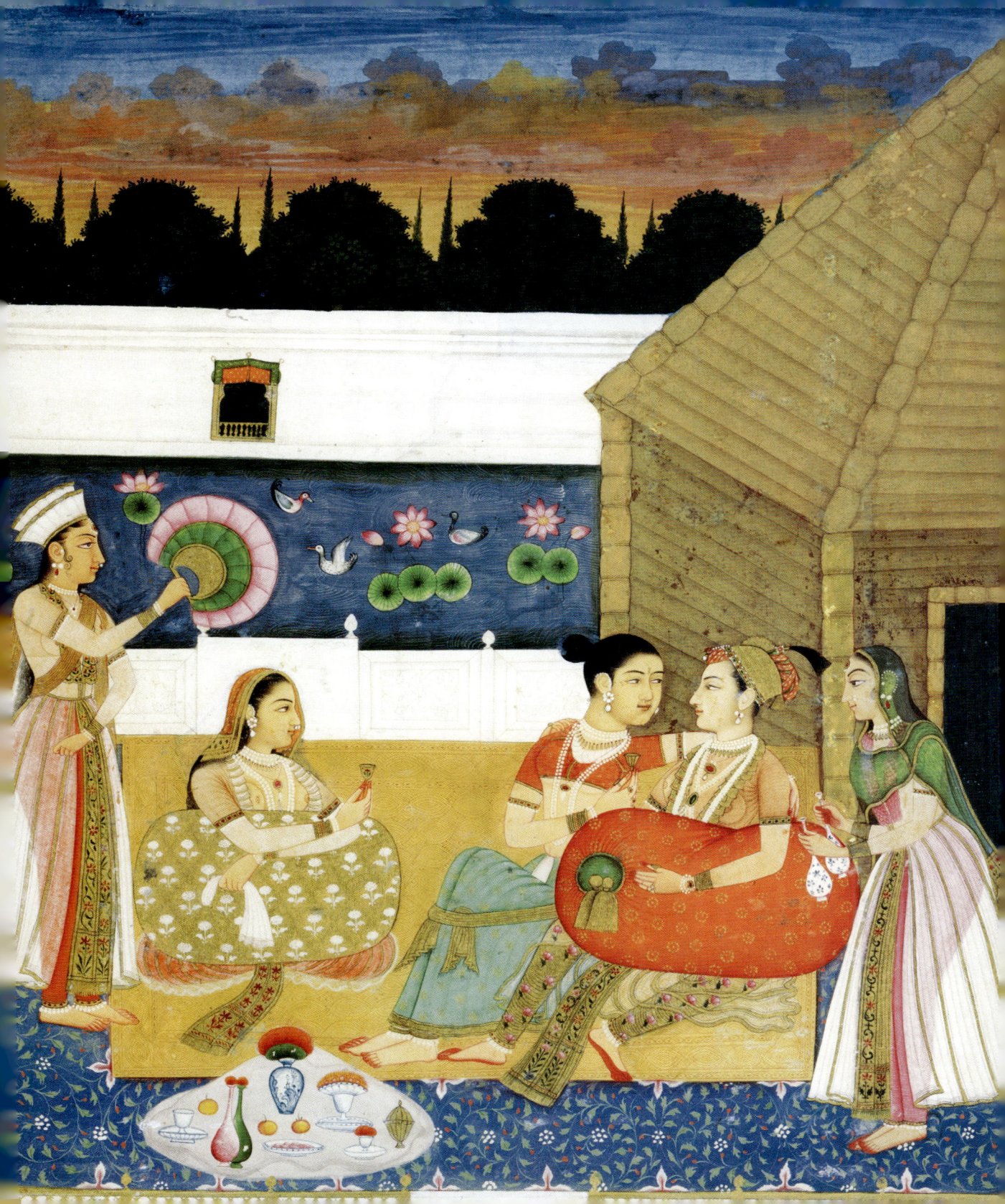

emotional and mental stimulation. Everything that helps enhance and heighten this sense of arousal and sexual awareness without actual penetration is known as foreplay.

Homosexual encounters too usually begin with foreplay and end in orgasm, but the pattern of lovemaking is much less rigid than the pattern of lovemaking between men and women. Not all encounters are necessarily homosexual: while some men want sex with other men as a permanent part of their lives, others are curious about male bodies and may experiment at some time of their lives; some feel equally attracted to men and women while other men enjoy looking at other men's bodies without desiring sexual contact. And these emotions are not restricted to men alone; women too feel and do these things with other women. Many men consider sex with other men to be liberating because there are no rules, there is much less pressure to perform and 'please' the woman as in a heterosexual relationship. For most men, foreplay may appear to be a waste of time because they understand each other's bodies so well. However, sensitive men who cuddle and kiss their partners and know how to engage in foreplay often find that they not only enjoy sex more, but also have an orgasm more often. The same holds true for women who say that there is a sense of unhurried pleasure and familiarity when it comes to making love to another women without having to put up with men who are inevitably in a hurry to get to the actual act. Women thus tend to lay a lot more emphasis on foreplay regarding it as not just essential, but an end in itself. Many women agree that physical affection is a much more significant expression of intimacy than sex and that they prefer intimacy to actual sex: kissing and embracing, sometimes takes precedence over the act. Both sexes believe that homoerotic relationships are more honest and straightforward, both physically and emotionally, and the lack of inhibition and pretense adds immensely to the sense of pleasure. The *Kama Sutra*, however, repeatedly says that reciprocity is absolutely essential to experience the joys of love. 'Every lover must reciprocate the beloved's gesture with equal intensity, a kiss for a kiss an embrace for an embrace. If there is no reciprocity, the beloved will feel dejected and consider the lover as a "stone-pillar", resulting in a highly unsatisfactory union.'

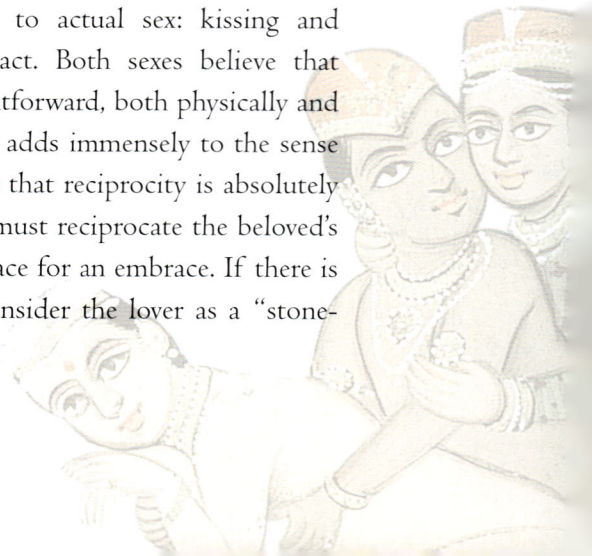

For both sexes, visual beauty is one of the chief components of sexual appeal, and a pleasing sight heighten tumescence; so the very first step in the seduction game is personal grooming. Vatsyayana lays a great deal of emphasis on hygiene and cleanliness to ensure that there are no offensive body odours, smelly mouths and other unwashed body parts. He recommends a rigid regime of washing and cleansing and application of scents and perfumes to the entire body. He says a man should 'bathe daily, anoint his body with oil every other day, apply a lathering substance every three days, get his head and face shaved every four days and the other parts of his body every five or ten days. All these things should be done without fail, and the sweat of the armpits should also be removed.' This is particularly true for homosexual men where hygiene should always be the first priority especially for those who engage in anal penetration. This done, the book says 'the man should paint his eyelids and below his eyes, colour his lips, chew things that give fragrance to the mouth.' On paying special attention to women, the *Kama Sutra* says: 'A woman being of a tender nature needs tender beginnings,' so a tender word, an intimate touch, a glass of wine to help shed inhibitions are all part of the recommended sixty-four ways through which passion can culminate in successful union.

Creating the right setting and environment, is the next step. Vatsyayana offers some very pragmatic advice on the venue and how to go about creating the right ambience for seduction: 'The house should be situated near water, and divided into different rooms for different purposes. It should be surrounded by a garden, and contain two rooms, an outer and an inner one. The outer room, suffused with rich perfumes, should contain a bed, soft, agreeable to the sight, covered with a clean white cloth, low in the middle part, having garlands and flowers strewn over it, a canopy above and two pillows, one at the top, another at the bottom. There should be also a sort of couch besides, and at the head of this a stool, on which should be placed fragrant ointments for the night, as well as flowers, pots containing collyrium and other fragrant substances, things used for perfuming the mouth, and the bark of the common citron tree. Near the couch, on the ground, there should be a pot for spitting, a box containing ornaments, a lute, a board for

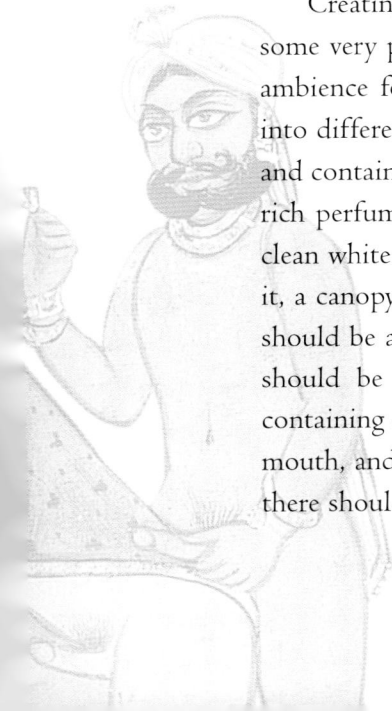

drawing, and a pot containing perfume, books, and garlands of the yellow amaranth flowers. Not far from the couch, and on the ground, there should be a round seat, a toy cart, and a board for playing with dice. Outside there should be cages of birds, and a separate place for spinning, carving and other such like diversions. In the garden there should be a whirling swing and a common swing, as also a bower of creepers covered with flowers, in which a raised parterre should be made for sitting.' This rather elaborate preparation holds good even today where much the same advice is given—bathtubs filled with rose petals, perfumed candles lit throughout the room, soft music, champagne flutes, chocolates, jasmine flowers and soft satin bed sheets.

Foreplay should be playful for unless there is humour, curiosity and liveliness in sex, it quickly loses its appeal. In these days of sexual overtness, flirting, the notion of catching one's eye across a room, and communicating desire through gestures may seem outdated, but many still thrill at an unexpected flash of interest across a room or an inviting gesture. Interpreting body language is an art that has never died out; to correctly interpret desire is indeed a skill that has to be acquired. The woman or man who wants to respond does so, according to the *Kama Sutra,* not overtly but with signs and gestures. The message that is sent out is implicit but without ambiguity: darting glances with a half-bent head, touching under some pretext, a feeling of being tongue-tied, playing with one's hair, adjusting one's clothes, aligning oneself towards the person you are interested in, leaning forward, gesticulating, playing with one's accessories, are all indications of interest. As is making eye contact, looking into someone's eyes just a fraction longer than necessary are all elements of the flirting process.

The human body is full of erogenous zones, places of great sexual sensitivity that are as, if not more, sensitive to touch and arousal than the obvious genital ones. What foreplay does is to help unravel these hidden mysteries. Flirting, kissing, touching, undressing, petting, cuddling are all-important for both partners to relax

*Facing page: Creating the right setting and environment is
an important pre-requisite in the game of love.*

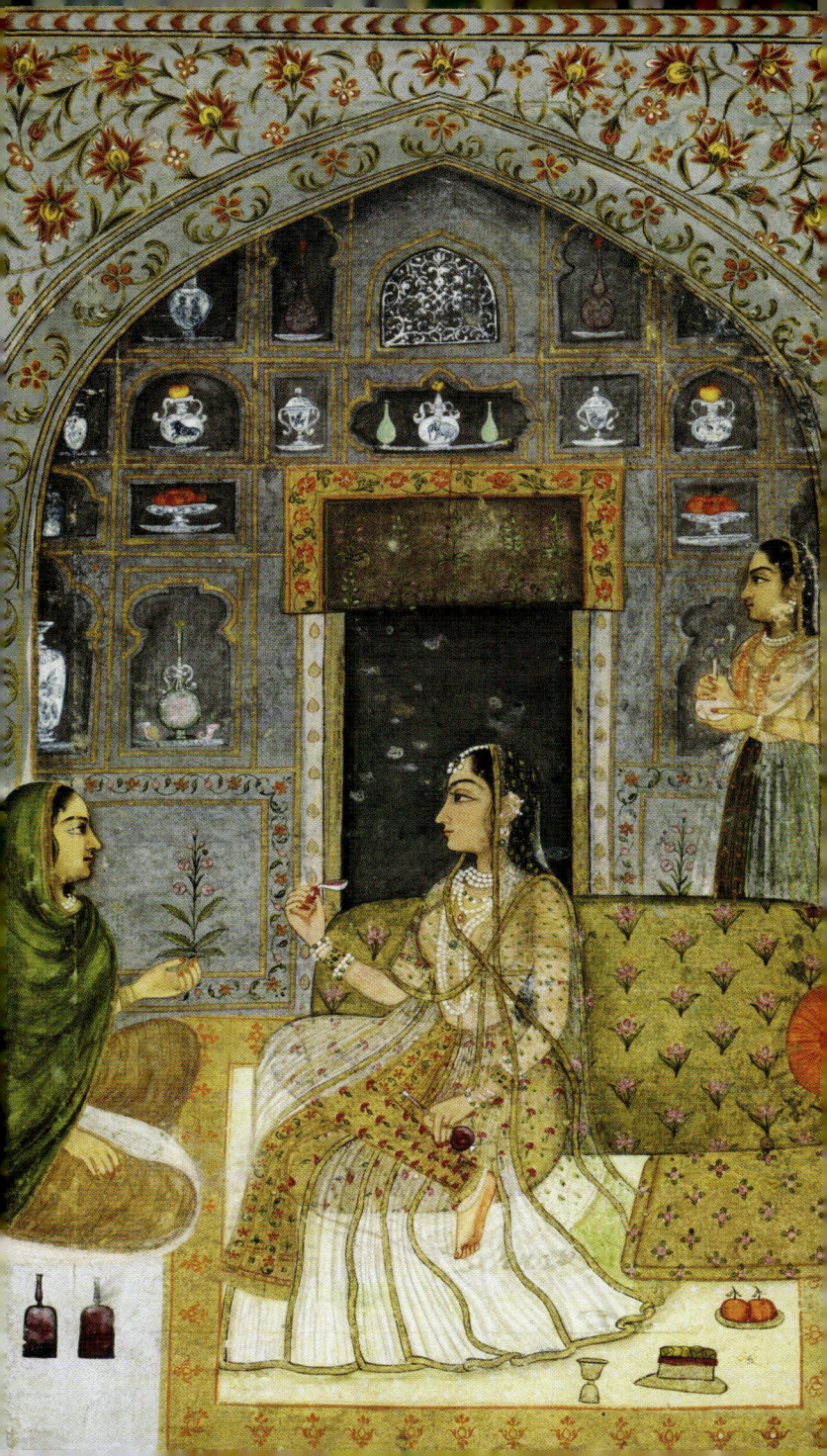

emotionally and physically and to become sexually aroused. Of all the five sense organs that come into play, the most responsive to stimuli is the sense of touch as the skin is acknowledged to be the body's largest sex organ. Tactility is a key factor in communicating desire, and touching provides a wonderful opportunity to explore the body's erogenous zones. Touching 'by accident' can have an extraordinary effect. Some *Kama Shastra* texts talk about how the hair on the arm stands on end, when a woman fleetingly touches her partner's arm. Even holding hands, caressing, hugging and embracing can become a highly erotic act of intimacy as can scratching the back, giving back rubs and oil massages. The *Kama Sutra* describes in detail how a man of the third sex who often works as a hairdresser and masseur, under the pretence of shampooing, embraces and draws towards himself the thighs of the man he is shampooing, and 'accidentally' touches his thighs and other body parts.

The ancient sages regarded these erogenous zones as substitutes for the genital organs and identified eight erogenous zones, which they divided into two sets of four. The first is associated with hair and includes the head, chin, armpits and the pubic area; the second consists of the mouth, nipples, genitals and the anus. Besides these there are secondary erogenous zones that include the palm of the hand, sole of the foot, fingertips, toes, knees, elbows, ears and the sacral region. The ancients also believed that the reaction of these body parts to stimuli varied with the phases of the moon. A 15th-century Sanskrit text called the *Smaradipika* has actually worked out a timetable, a chart if you will, that gives in great detail specific parts of the body that are best stimulated according to the waxing and waning moon. Briefly, according to the book: 'The places where passion resides in women during the *shuklapaksh* or the bright fortnight; that is passion can be aroused by: Pressing the toe of the feet on the 1st day of the waxing moon makes it an erogenous zone, scratching the vulva with one's fingernails on the 3rd day, rubbing the navel on the 8th day,' and so on. The *Kama Sutra* refers to the use of 'elephant trunks', that is, the first and fourth fingers being turned down into the palm and joined together, and the middle finger then being used for penetration imitating an elephant's trunk. The elephant trunk could also refer to the use of artificial instruments like dildos and modern-day vibrators.

Besides using the hand, the tongue too can play a vital role in the game of arousal. Licking with the tongue and exploring the entire length of each other's bodies can be a delicious form of foreplay. Fingers too can be used creatively in adventurous pleasuring: caressing the different parts of the body, kissing the hand tenderly, massaging the body with aromatic oils are all highly erotic. Exploring the vagina with the fingers is also an intimate form of foreplay. Many women enjoy the sensation of fingers deep inside their vagina, caressing the cervix and stimulating the g-spot, which leads to instantaneous release.

Intimate contact is of two kinds—external and internal. External contact involves fondling, caressing, kissing, touching…without actual intercourse. With increasing intimacy, an external contact is converted into an internal one during which no barriers exist. Foreplay, however, need not necessarily always lead to sex. Especially women say that they prefer intimacy to actual sex: kissing, embracing, exploring with the tongue all take precedence over the act itself as these portray a caring relationship rather than one of instant gratification. This is particularly true for lesbian women who, eschewing the roughness and urgency often exhibited by men, tend to linger over one another cherishing the moments of shared intimacy. Men, on the other hand, tend to eschew foreplay, but the *Kama Sutra* guides both men and women to sensually and erotically experience intimacy without intercourse.

Embracing

Embracing is the very first stage of physical intimacy and believed to have four distinct stages—touching, pulling, rubbing and pressing hard. First the partners touch each other lovingly and move closer in the next stage. Once their bodies come into contact, the lovers begin to touch, caress and stroke each other and as desire mounts, both press hard against each other as a prelude to intercourse. There are according to the *Kama Sutra* eight kinds of embraces with four additional ones like the embrace of the thighs, the embrace of the *jaghana* (the part of the body from the navel downwards to the thighs), the embrace of the breasts and the embrace of the forehead in which the lovers touch the mouth, eyes and the forehead of the other with their own. Those described in the *Kama Sutra* often have quaint names but rather illustrate the point: the *jataveshtitaka*, or the twining of a creeper where a woman clings to another as a creeper twines round a tree, bending her head while slightly making the sound *'sut sut'*; the *vrikshadhirudhaka* or the climbing of a tree; the *tila-tandulaka*, or the mixture of sesame seeds with rice is when lovers lying on a bed.

Kissing

Kissing which is a highly satisfying pleasure in itself can be extremely sensuous and need not be restricted to the mouth. Every part of the body should be kissed and explored; in fact according to the *Kama Sutra*, no position is worthwhile unless it facilitates kissing. The most ancient Indian texts on erotology list the parts of the body that are particularly sensitive to being kissed: the forehead, cheeks, eyes, breasts, nipples, lips, and the vulva. Each type of kiss is also given a name: The Kiss That Kindles Love, The Clasping Kiss, The Bent Kiss, The Sucking Kiss, among many others. The Surprise Kiss catches the lover unawares, when he's busy, occupied, working or even asleep, while The Vacuum Kiss is a playful and flirtatious kiss. The most sensuous of these is The Butterfly Kiss done by fluttering one's eye lashes on your lover's skin and is believed to be highly erotic when done on the penis. Since much of lesbian sex is foreplay, kissing assumes a great deal of importance here. Licking, sucking the upper chest and collarbone area, running the tongue over the breasts, waistline, navel and stomach, swirling the tongue on the nipples, nibbling the nipples are all guaranteed to result in multiple orgasms for both women.

Facing page: Women prefer acts of intimacy: kissing, embracing, exploring bodies all take precedence over the actual act of sex.

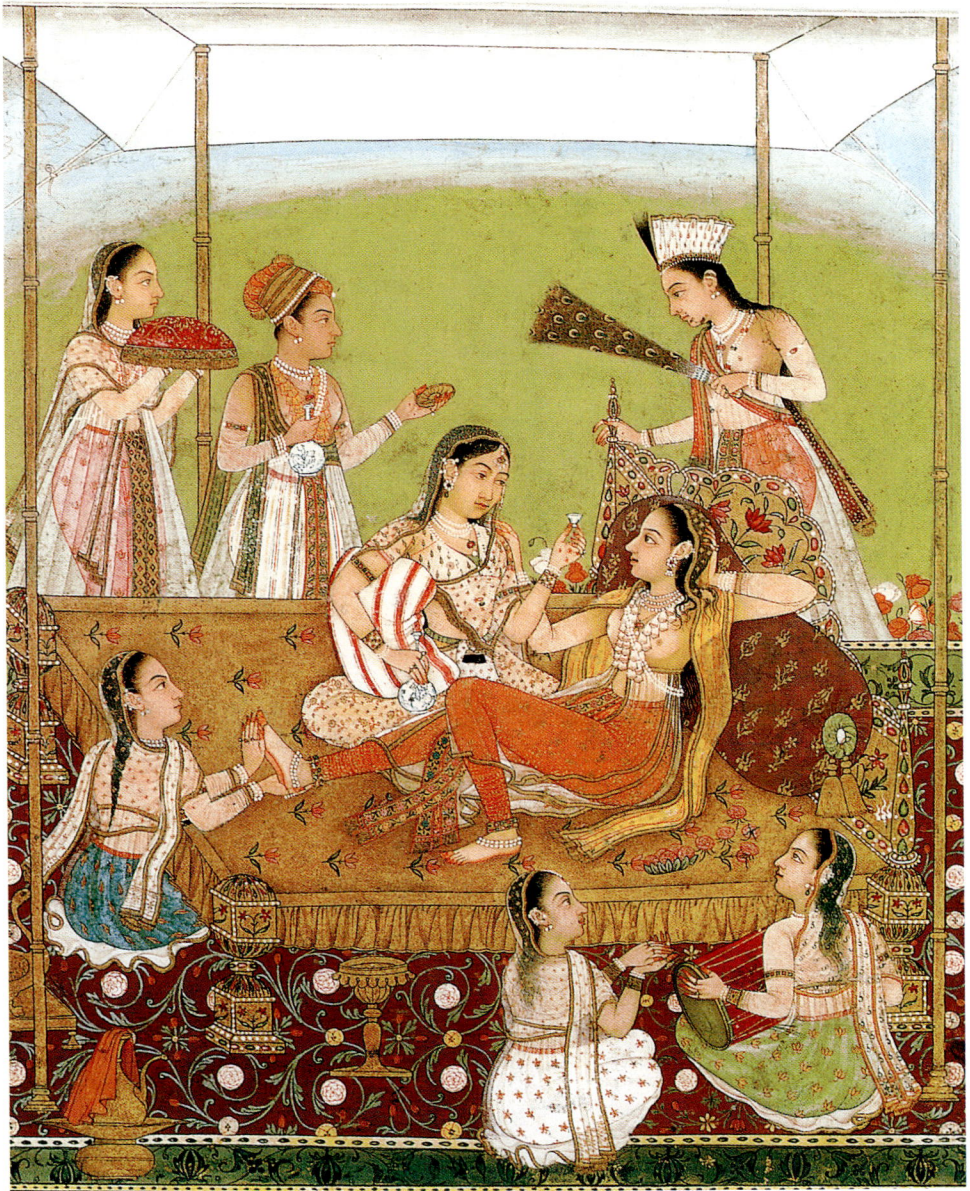

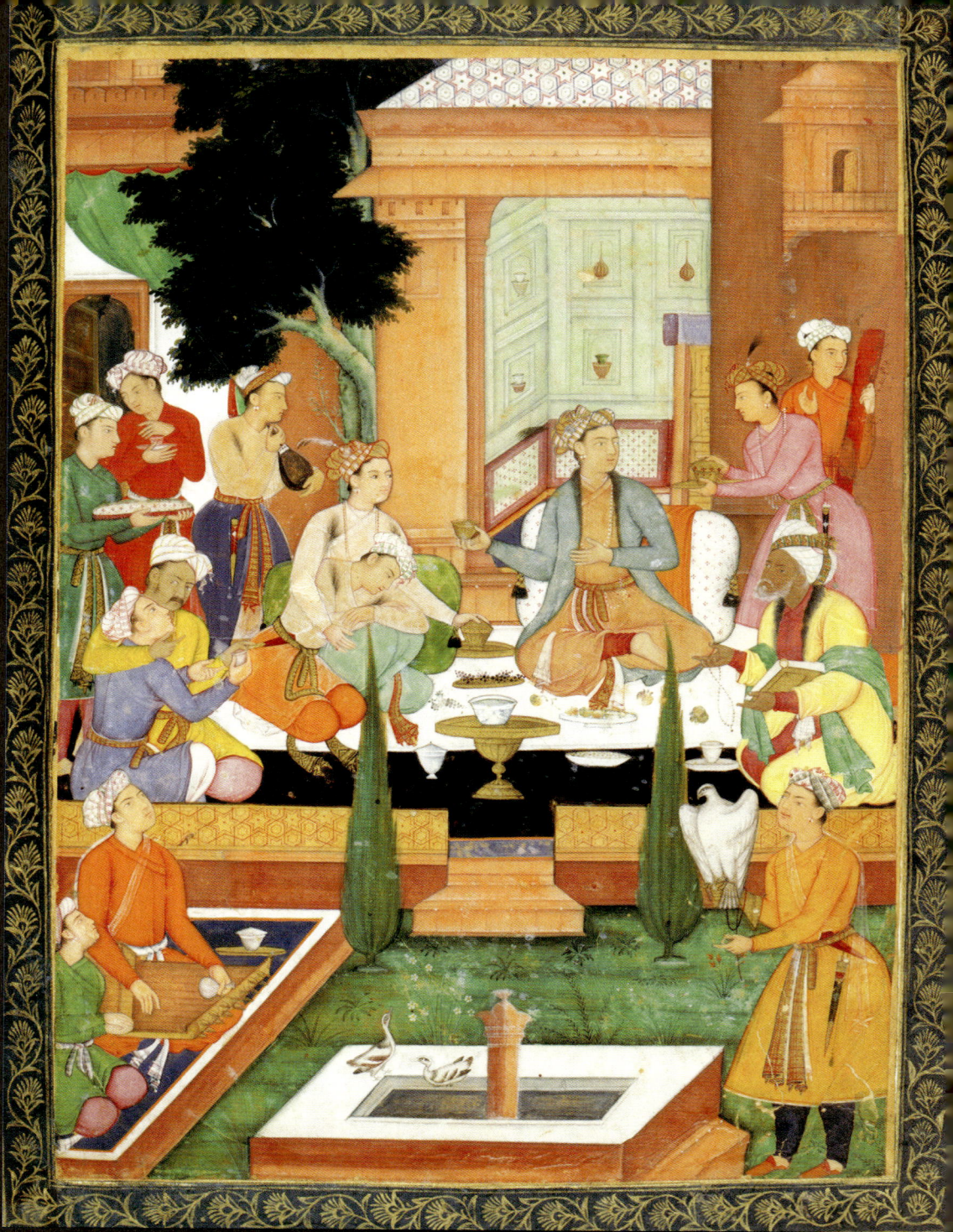

Nail Marks

While kissing kindles the fire of love, scratching adds fuel to keep the fire of passion burning. When desire heightens automatically both partners attain the requisite degree of excitement and automatically leave marks on each other's bodies. Nail marks can be used on the armpits, breasts, neck, back, thighs, vagina but care must be taken not to inflict lasting or painful marks. Nail marks are like a badge of honour to be proudly displayed in remembrance of the night of passion. Similarly, biting is also said to be an indication of the intensity of passion, though biting must be done in a manner so as not to leave permanent marks. Nibbling the neck, breasts and thighs are said to be highly exciting. While hitting may seem rather archaic and even barbaric today most *Kama Shastra* texts recommend both of them. Hitting the partner and simultaneously making sibilating sounds are believed to be explicit ways of showing the level of excitement. Sibilation usually accompanies hitting, where associated sounds like hissing, sighing, are produced as the sense of sound heightens passion. Ancient texts recommend that women keep repeating '*sut*' '*sut*' during the act of intercourse.

Foreplay doesn't end with intercourse or orgasm as the most precious moments in a relationship come soon after making love. The *Kama Sutra* reminds us that it is impolite to sleep too soon: 'Those things that increase passion should be done first, and those for amusement should be done afterward.' It recommends embracing and kissing after intercourse, and after cleaning and bathing, spending time with each other by talking, playing games, drinking and partaking of good foods.

The *Kama Sutra* continues to speak to us from a distant past giving pragmatic advice that remains relevant to this day. This text places a great deal of importance on balance and the need to place a partner's need before one's own. It recognizes the fact that women take more time to get aroused and recommends foreplay especially in the case of lesbians. As with heterosexual couples, initiating

Facing page: Wooing is a lesson for a lifetime, to be learnt and redefined at various stages of every relationship.

intercourse before both partners are equally ready will invariably lead to discontentment and unhappiness. Inevitably too, intercourse where there is no mutual desire, lasts only a few minutes, which makes it more than evident why the *Kama Sutra* so thoroughly addresses the need for multiple forms of love play.

So wooing a partner has to continue well after the initial flush of love has been consummated because skill and patience is required to recapture those moments of ecstasy. 'Wooing is a lesson for a lifetime, to be learnt and redefined at various stages of every relationship.' Great sex is so much more than bodies rubbing together, requiring trust, intimacy, communication, grace as well as etiquette. So the *Kama Sutra* recommends that the ideal of romance be maintained throughout the game of love, which requires relentless patience and persistence. The *Kama Sutra* teaches us how to make love an art and rekindle desire. As one commentary on the text succinctly puts it, 'It teaches you the very important lesson that sex is not an afterthought at the end of your day.'

Facing page: Recognizing that women take longer to get aroused, foreplay is of utmost importance and recommended.
Following pages 82-83: During the long absence of their menfolk, women in zenanas often pleasured each other.

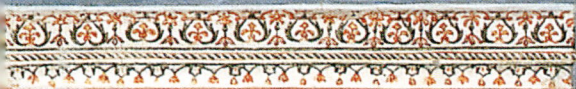

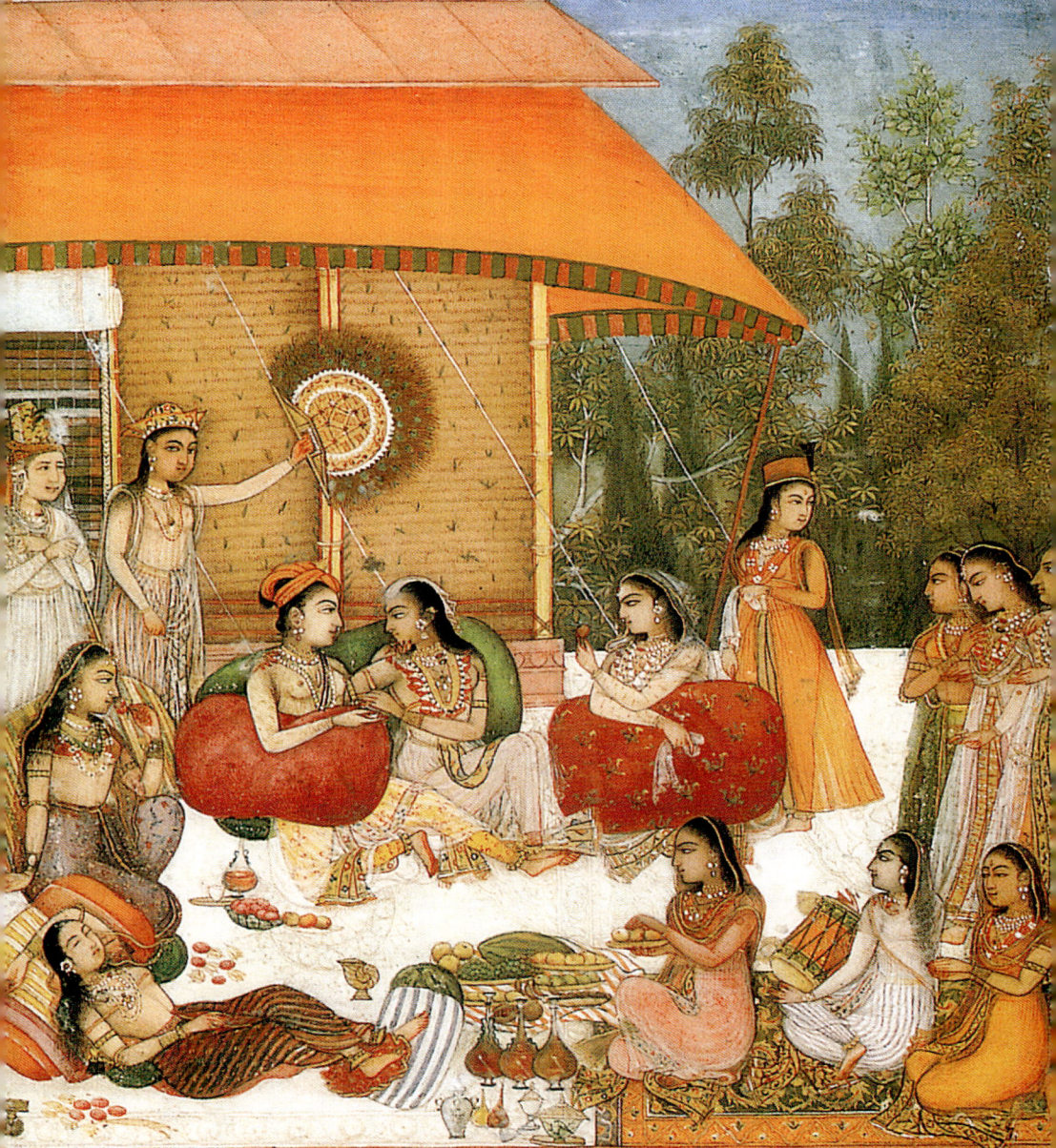

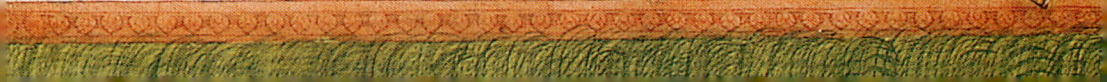

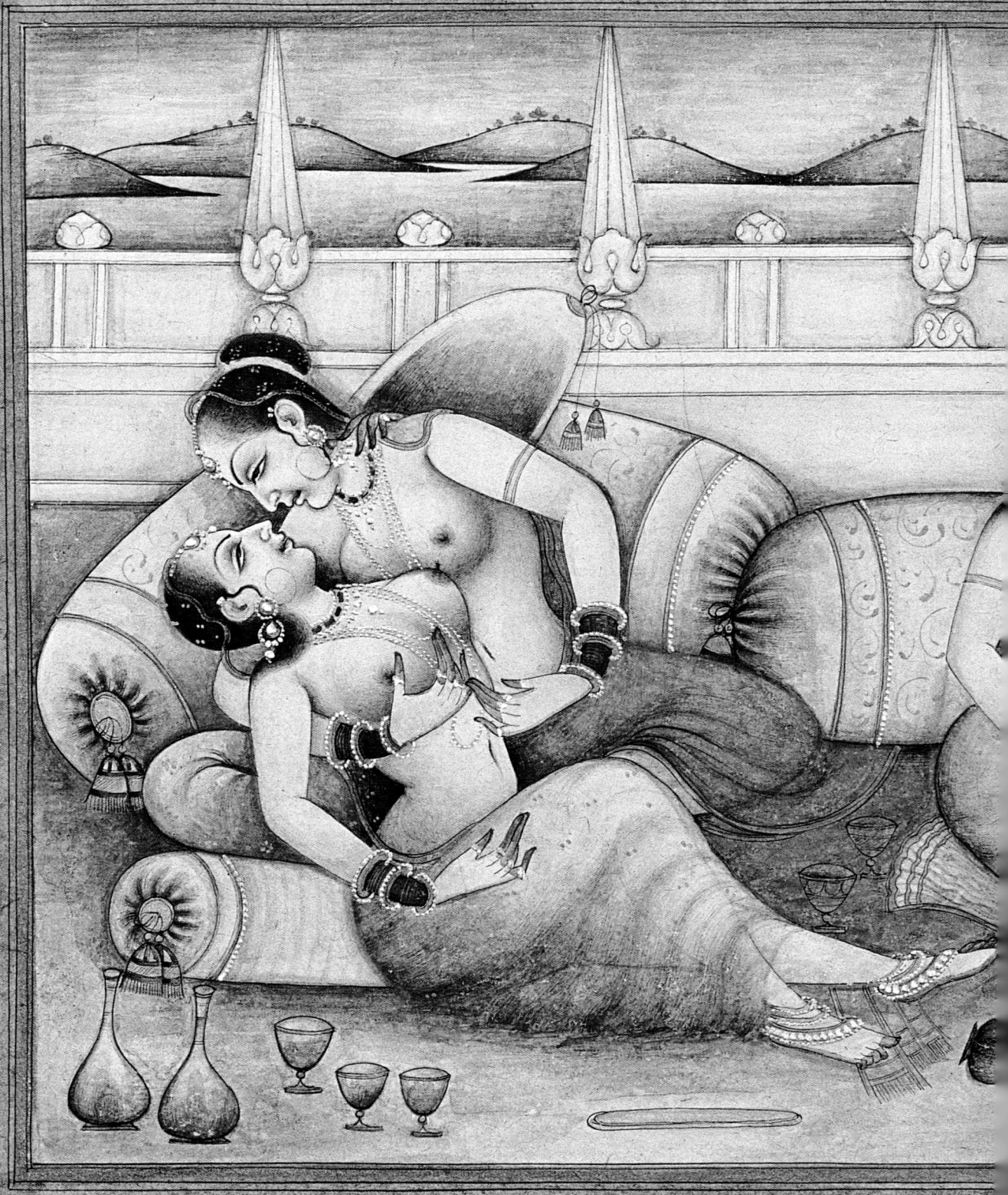

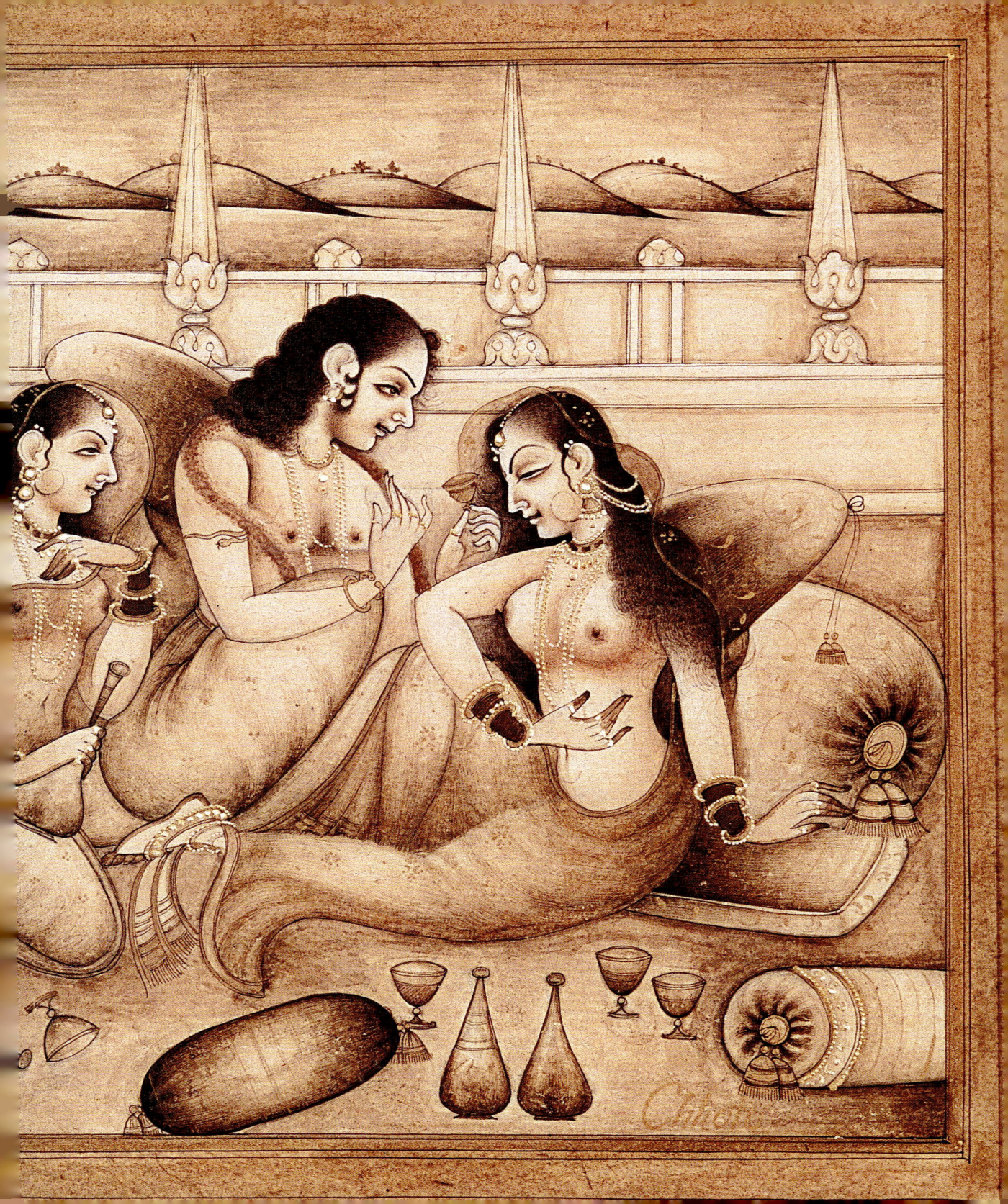

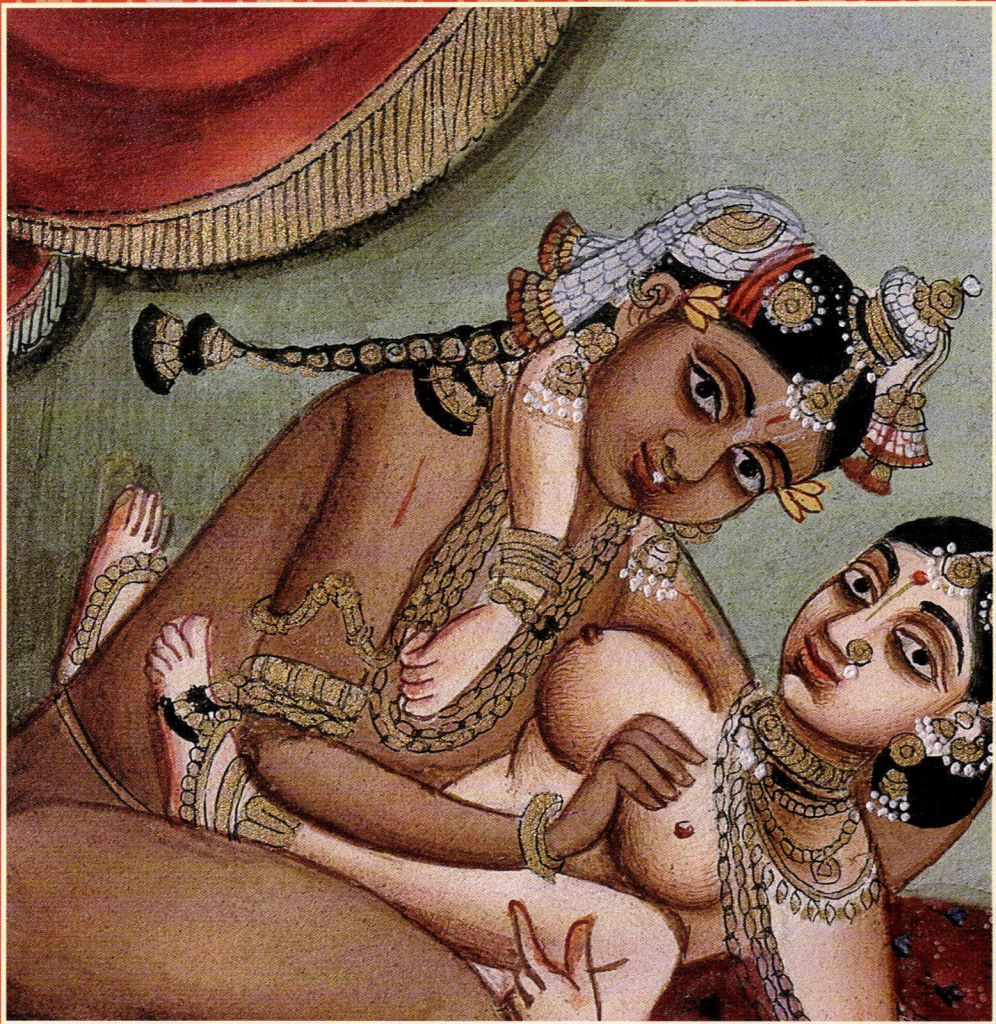

Postures

The *Kama Sutra* was first introduced to the world by Sir Francis Richard Burton who was a famous Victorian orientalist and traveller. On his return to England from India he along with several friends founded the London Anthropological Society, that brought out a periodical called *Anthropologia* which became instrumental in educating the Western world about the diversity of human sexual behaviour: 'My motive was to supply travellers with an organ that would rescue their observations from the outer darkness of manuscripts, and print their curious information on social and sexual matters,' wrote Burton. He also co-founded the Kama Shastra Society, a small and highly secretive organization that privately published the

Kama Sutra (in 1883) and the *Ananga Ranga* (in 1885), the first ancient Hindu treatises on the art of love to be translated into the English language. Interestingly they could not be 'officially' published in English until the mid 1960s, following a landmark court case.

The *Kama Sutra* has become the world's foremost treatise on ancient sexuality. Bolstered by erotic miniature paintings that depict the sixty-four postures, the book has probably become more voyeuristic than a work worthy of study. But the illustrations belie its true worth, for the *Kama Sutra* continues to speak to us. Its modernity and wisdom appear more appropriate today than ever before as does its inclusiveness and acceptance of all aspects of sexual life. Twenty centuries ago, Vatsyayana had come to the very sophisticated conclusion that unequal partnerships lead to unfulfilled passions that in turn lead to unhappiness and discontentment. The solution, according to him, was to strike the right balance between all the human urges: physical, emotional, intellectual, social, sexual as well as spiritual. Compatibility was a key factor and he surmised that to get maximum pleasure, partners had to suit each other in every respect, be it in temperament, the extent of passion, their physiques right down to even the size of their genital organs. With a comprehensive understanding of inter-personal relationships, the *Kama Sutra* offers some very urbane insights for satisfactory sex and ways to prevent tedium from setting in between couples. 'The chief reason for separation is the desire for varied pleasures and the monotony that follows possession. Monotony begets satiety, and satiety distaste for congress, and soon one or the other yields to temptation.' Dependency created by habit has to be first broken as this provides a false sense of security and restricts the entire ways of life and conscious choices. Of all habits, sexual habits are indeed the most restrictive. The *Kama Sutra* says: 'Love resulting from the constant and continual performance of an act is called love acquired by habit.'

The solution was to provide variety—in the place of making love, postures, styles, surroundings—all considered necessary, and not only to combat monotony.

While the *Kama Sutra* describes sixty-four postures, every man and woman knows that more than technique, what is required for a fulfilling encounter is passion. A performance remains just that if acted out without the tenderness and compassion that drives all human emotion: when desire overwhelms the body and spirits soar high, when every caress, touch, eye contact, whisper and position comes alive and is savoured. So, gymnastics in bed is not the endgame, but a means to explore every avenue to enhance sensation rather than slip into boredom and

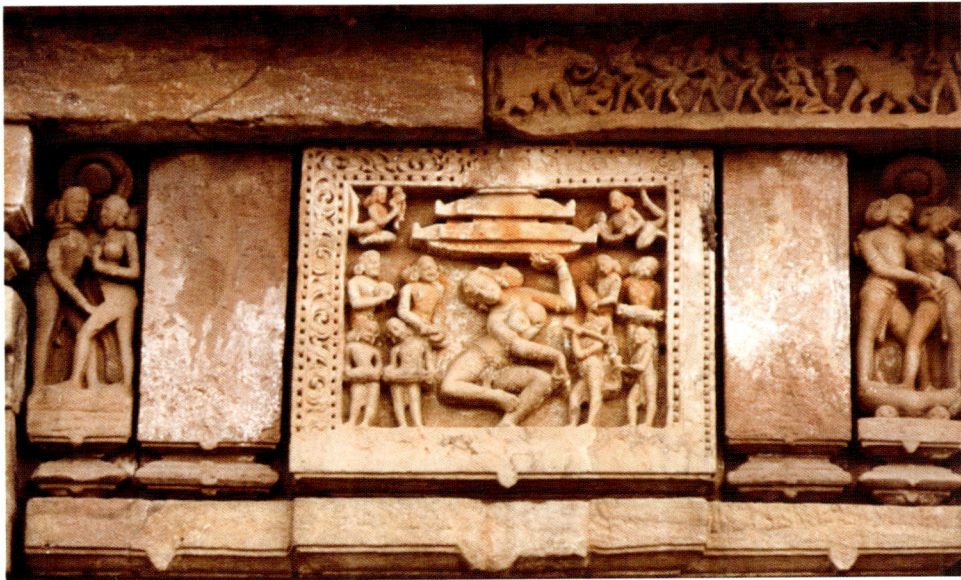

repugnance. The *Kama Sutra* opens up a world of sexual choreography and technique that can be learned methodically and from whose knowledge comes new insight—a way to rediscover passion and intimacy.

The purpose of these detailed descriptions is to ensure that both women and men understand the complexities involved in intimacy. However, establishing sensual connections needs personal maturity, attentiveness and disciplining the

Establishing sensual connections needs maturity, attentiveness and disciplining the mind as well as the body.

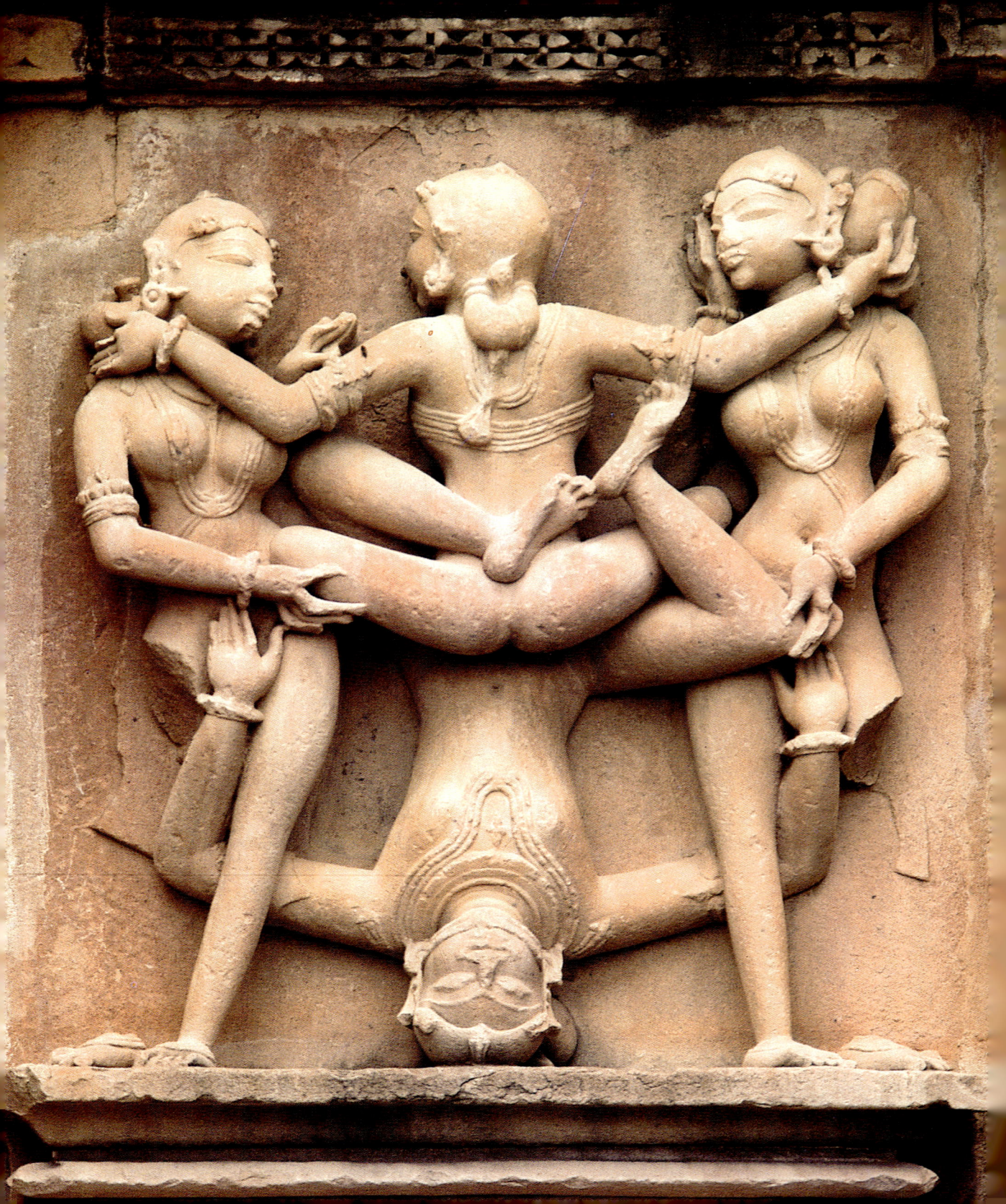

mind as well as the body. The postures recommended in the text were derived from Patanjali's famous *Yoga Shastras* and were meant not just to keep the body supple but also to develop the mind. These *asanas* were 'attitudes' designed to make the body strong and flexible, balanced and graceful, healthy and fit, as well as increase the body's reservoir of energy. The positions described, however, went beyond mere contortions, and were based on scientific classifications that analysed which partners would be best suited for maximizing pleasure. With a word of caution and humour though, Vatsyayana warns that while some positions are basic enough, others are decidedly acrobatic and should not be attempted until one is extremely fit and supple.

Considering that making love was a sin only if done badly, books of sexual wisdom such as the *Kama Sutra*, *Ananga Ranga*, *Smaradipika*, *Ratirahasya* or even the *Perfumed Garden* and the *Tao*, offer sensible and practical advice or how to enhance sexual pleasure. The *Ananga Ranga* by Kalyana Malla (late 15th or early 16th century), for example, was written to prevent sexual tedium from setting in. It describes various groups of lovemaking positions such as the *uttana-bandha* (supine positions with the man on top), the *tiryak-bandha* (side-by-side positions), the *upavishta* (sitting positions), and the *purushayita-bandha* (woman-on-top positions). The late 15th-century *Perfumed Garden* written for a male-dominated North African-Arabic culture offers ample and often evocative instruction on what a man could do. The *Tao*, a collection of ancient Chinese wisdom, predates the *Kama Sutra* and lays emphasis on the fact that sexual energy can be used to improve health, harmonize relationships, and lead to spiritual realization. In the *Tao* the author describes twenty-six positions for lovemaking such as Intimate Union (man-on-top), the Unicorn's Horn (woman-on-top), Close Attachment (side-by-side), and the Fish Sunning Itself (rear entry), among others.

Facing page: Postures are designed to make the body strong, supple and flexible for maximizing pleasure.

Positions

Sexual positions refer to the different ways in which couples physically position themselves for intercourse. Theoretically there can be countless positions, but in fact, most are variations on less than half a dozen basic postures. Popular belief among heterosexual couples is that the man-on-top position is the only normal and acceptable coital position; it is also believed that there are scores of sexual positions and that no one may be deemed a competent lover until he or she has mastered them all. There is a further myth that suggests that the more physically challenging the position, the greater the sexual satisfaction. None of these myths are of course true. Competence in lovemaking is measured by fulfillment and not by the extent of one's sexual repertoire.

So although the *Kama Sutra* lists sixty-four positions, in most sexual encounters, the most common sexual positions are only five: man-on-top, woman-on-top, side-by-side, rear-entry, anal and oral intercourse performed lying down, sitting, standing, kneeling, or a combination of all this.

The man-on-top is the most common position and is also known as the missionary position named so after the 19th-century Christian missionaries who encouraged their converts to abandon their so-called 'animal' positions in favour of the man-on-top position. In the woman-on-top position the man lies on his back and the woman lowers herself onto his erect penis and can thus regulate the depth of penetration of the penis and the rate of thrusting. This position also allows for maximal indirect stimulation and some women reach orgasm more easily when they are on top. This is known as the Reversal of Roles in the *Kama Sutra* and is described as a position adapted by women who sometimes behave as men. Described rather picturesquely as the Swing *(Dola)*, Pair of Tongs and the Spinning Top, these are positions that can be adapted just as easily by women making love to other women.

Facing page: When a man enjoys many women at the same time,
it is called the 'congress of a herd of cows'.

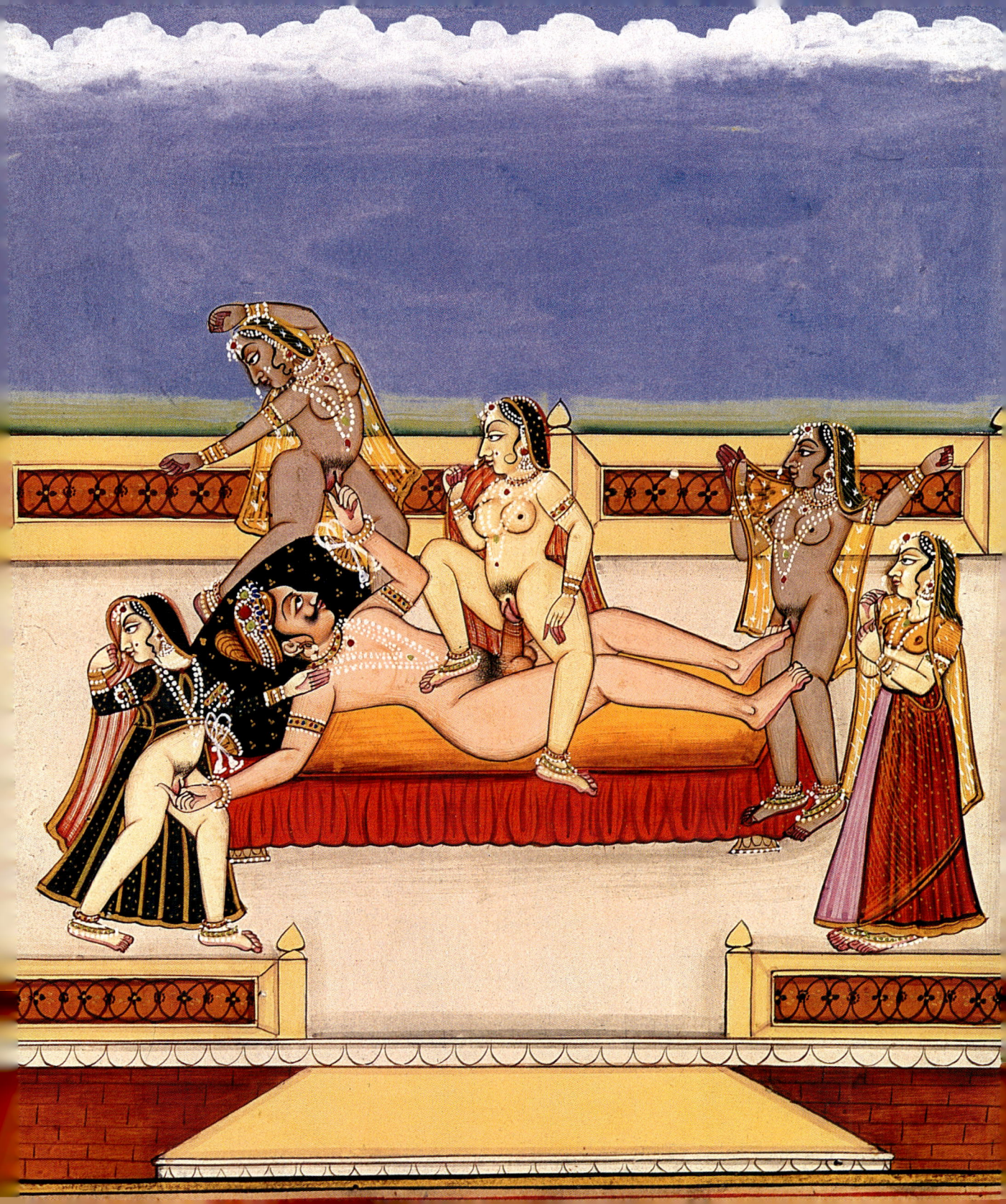

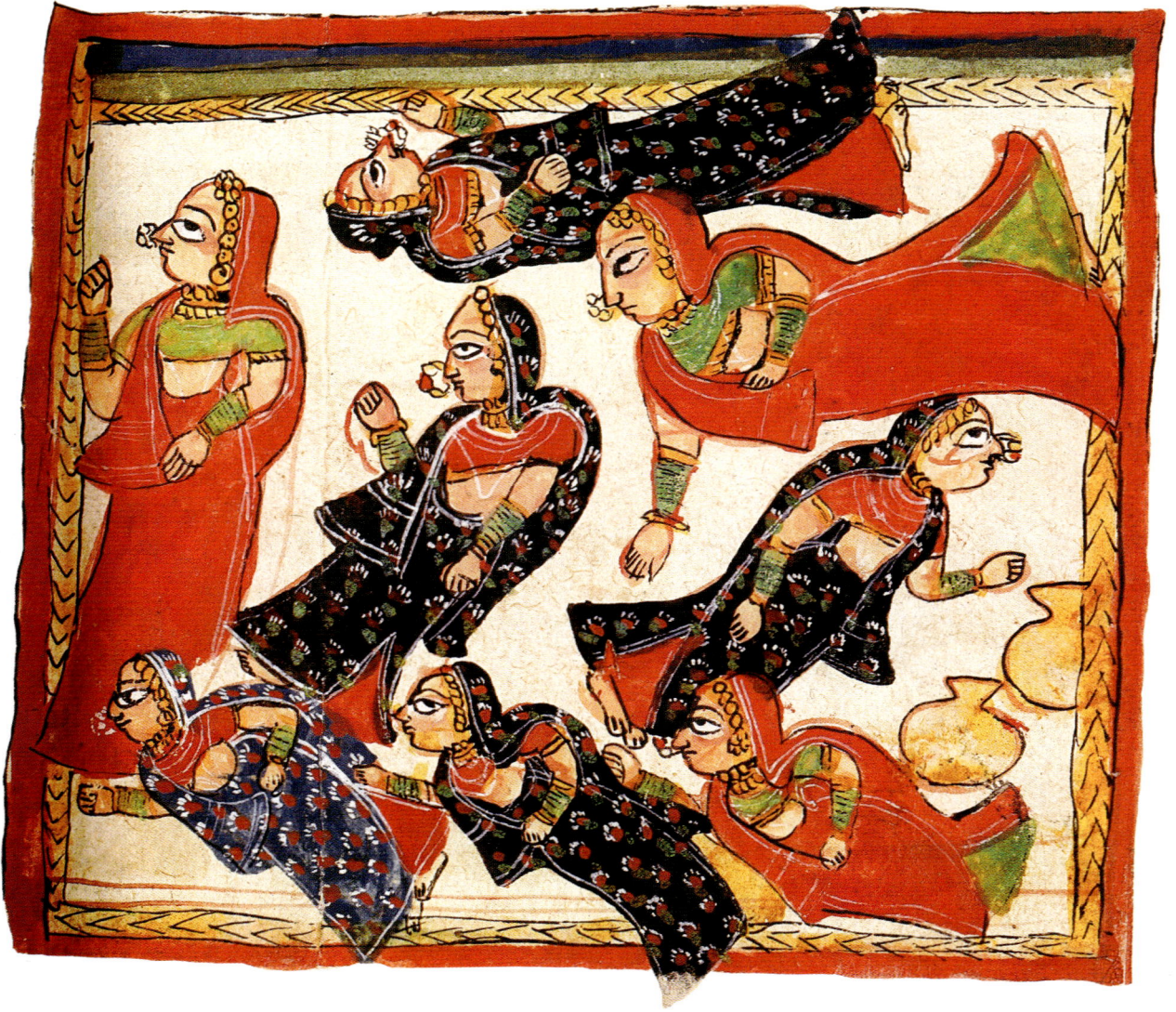

Female friends add a quaint charm to a couple's courtship

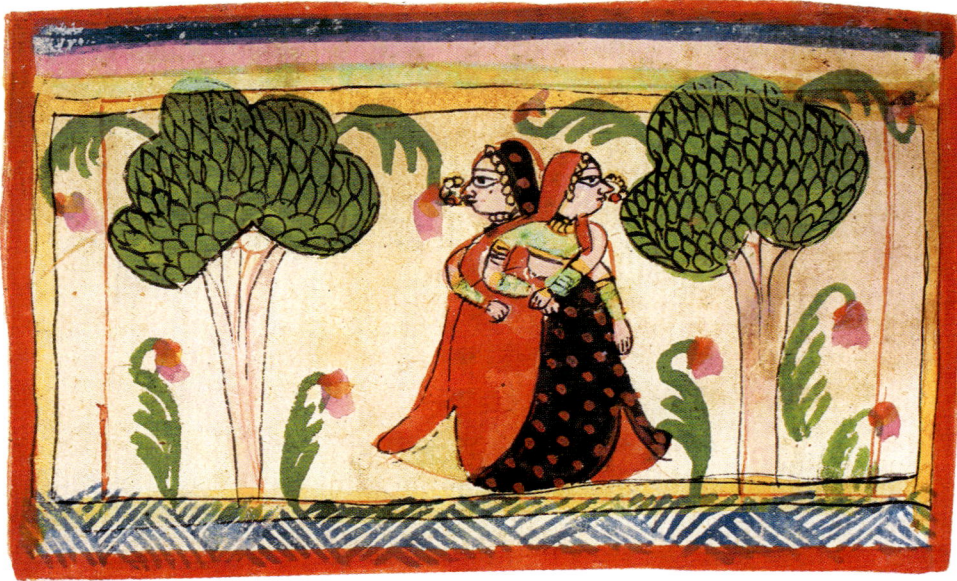

The side-by-side position is a position in which the partners have intercourse lying on their sides facing each other. Deep pelvic thrusting is difficult when a couple is side by side; on the other hand, both partners' hands are free to caress each other and the face-to- face position allows them to kiss. The *Kama Sutra* recommends that the man lie to the left and the woman to the right, but as with everything else personal preferences are what matters.

Rear entry intercourse is when the man's penis enters the woman's vagina when she has her back to him. It is not the same as anal intercourse, which is intercourse with a man's penis inserted in his partner's rectum. Rear entry intercourse can be done with the woman standing but bending over and supporting herself, or with the woman on her hands and knees and the man kneeling behind her (commonly known as doggy style). Rear entry allows for deep penetration and vigorous pushing and the man's hands are free to caress the woman and he can reach her clitoris easily.

The *Kama Sutra* also offers detailed positions for oral and anal intercourse, which, though not recommended are also explored as is the use of artificial aids

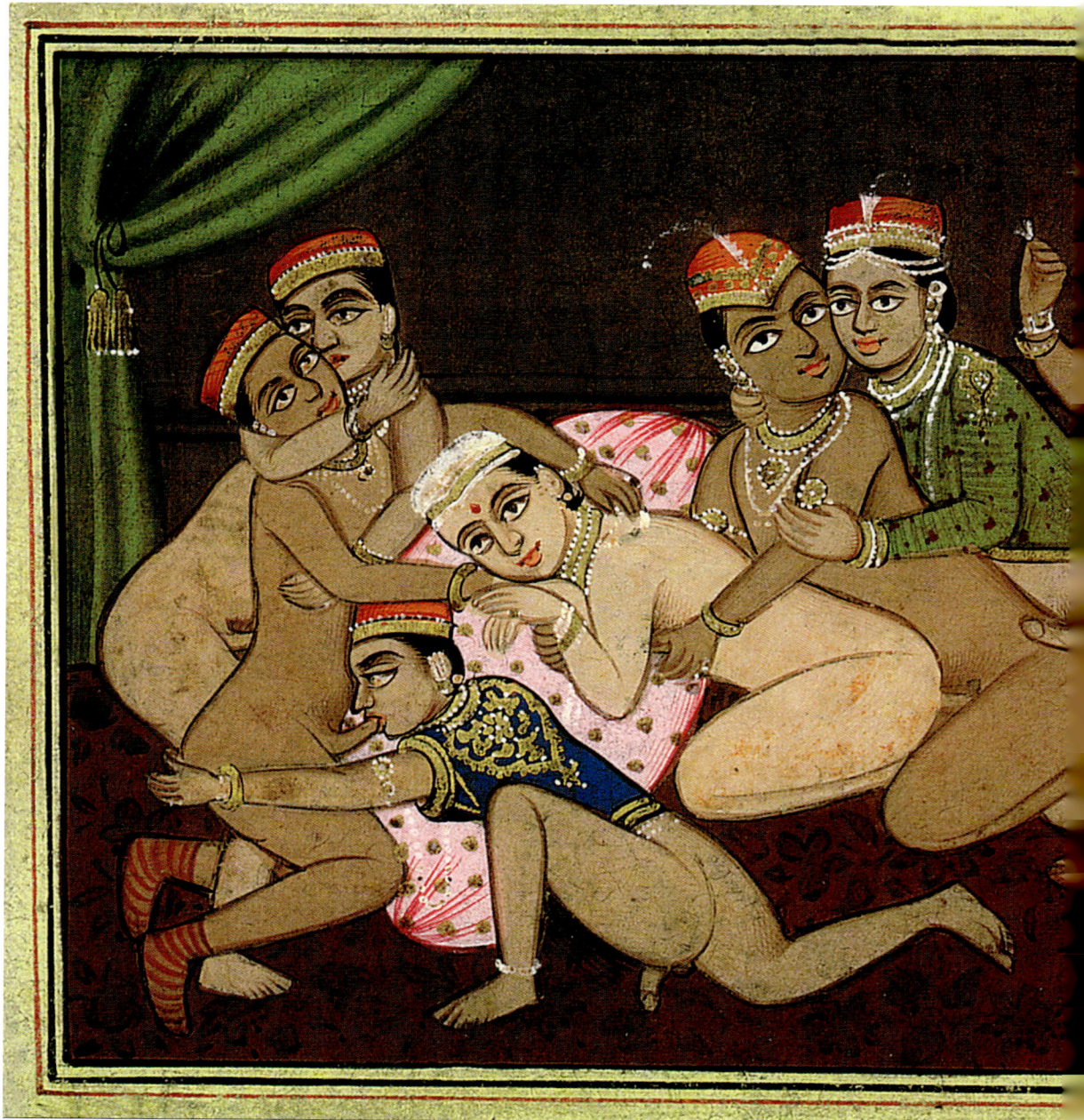

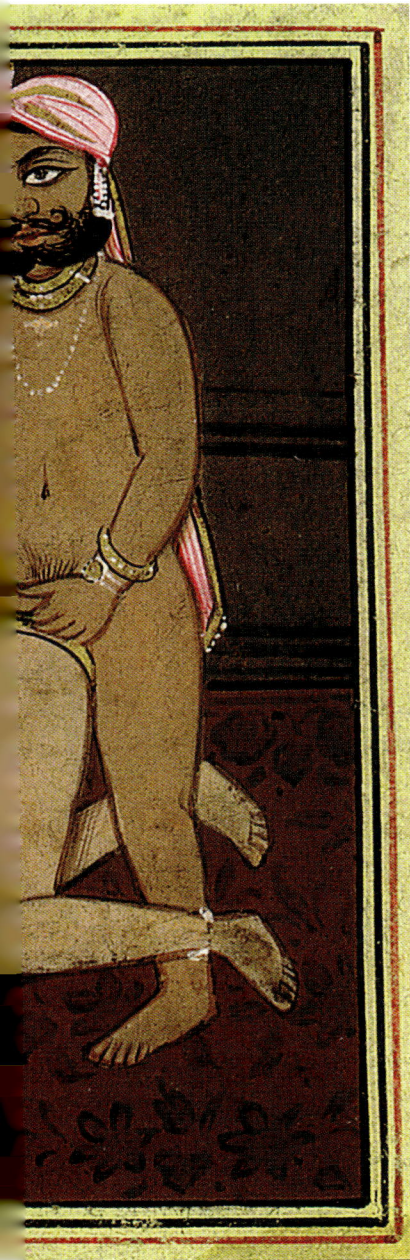

such as dildos. With the exception of coitus, sexual positions for gay and lesbian couples do not differ much from those of heterosexual couples, since the vast array of sexual positions that same-sex or opposite-sex couples may use remains basically the same.

Gay men may engage in anal intercourse more often than heterosexual couples and gay women may be more likely to introduce sexual aids into their lovemaking. The acceptance of homosexual tendencies in these texts is a reflection of the sophistication and social ability of the times to be adaptive as well as tolerant. Vedic sages understood that some humans do not bear the precise socio-sexual imprint that society expects and demands of them. This did and continues to often result in them hiding their true sexual profiles by either imitating or accepting specified gender-specific roles. Many men and women, while living within the confines of these roles, yearn to live by their own sexual proclivities.

Whatever be one's sexual preference, the need to be loved and the act of physical intimacy as an expression of that love is a universal human quality and the *Kama Sutra* only attempts to help by enumerating these different positions and techniques as a means of achieving that basic fulfilment.

The *Kama Sutra* suggests many sitting, lying down, standing and side-by-side positions. Some of these are listed below:

Homosexual love was dominant in many cultures of the world.

Lying Down Positions

A primary position when lying down, this is known as Indrani after
Lord Indra's wife; this position is specially loved by young
and supple girls but takes a lot of practice:

SHE CUPS AND LIFTS HER BUTTOCKS WITH HER PALMS,
SPREADS WIDE HER THIGHS, AND DIGS IN HER HEELS BESIDES HER HIPS,
WHILE YOU CARESS HER BREASTS:
THIS IS *UTPHALLAKA* (THE FLOWER IN BLOOM).

GRASPING THE ANKLES OF THE ROUND-HIPPED WOMAN,
WHOSE BUTTOCKS ARE LIKE TWO RIPE GOURDS,
RAISE HER BEAUTIFUL THIGHS AND SPREAD THE THIGH-JOINTS WIDELY.
FULL OF DESIRE, SAYING SWEET WORDS,
APPROACH HER WITH YOUR BODY STIFF AS A POLE
AND DRIVE STRAIGHT FORWARD
TO PIERCE HER LOTUS AND JOIN YOUR LIMBS:
EXPERTS CALL IT *MADANDHVAJA* (THE FLAG OF CUPID).

CATCH HOLD OF HER TWO FEET,
RAISING THEM TILL THEY PRESS UPON HER BREASTS
AND HER LEGS FORM A ROUGH CIRCLE.
CLASP HER NECK AND MAKE LOVE TO HER:
THIS IS *RATISUNDARA* (APHRODITE'S DELIGHT).

LIFT THE LADY'S FEET UNTIL HER SOLES LIE PERFECTLY PARALLEL,
ONE TO EACH SIDE OF HER SLENDER THROAT,
CUP HER BREASTS AND ENJOY HER:
THIS TECHNIQUE IS *UTHKANTA* (THROAT-HIGH).

⁂

YOUR LOVELY WIFE, LYING ON THE BED,
GRASPS HER OWN FEET
AND DRAWS THEM UP UNTIL THEY REACH HER HAIR;
YOU CATCH HER BREASTS AND MAKE LOVE:
THIS IS *VYOMAPADA* (SKY-FOOT).

⁂

THE ROUND-THIGHED WOMAN ON THE BED
GRASPS HER ANKLES AND RAISES HIGH HER LOTUS FEET;
YOU STRIKE HER TO THE ROOT, KISSING
AND SLAPPING OPEN-PALMED BETWEEN HER BREASTS:
THIS IS *MARKATA* (THE MONKEY).

⁂

SHE LIES FLAT ON HER BACK,
YOU SIT BETWEEN HER PARTED KNEES, RAISE THEM,
HOOK HER FEET OVER YOUR THIGHS,
CATCH HOLD OF HER BREASTS, AND ENJOY HER:
THIS IS *MANMATHPRIYA* (DEAR TO CUPID)

Seated Positions

SEATED, MOUTH-TO-MOUTH, ARMS AGAINST ARMS,
THIGHS AGAINST THIGHS: THIS IS *KAURMA* (THE TORTOISE).

IF THE LOVERS' THIGHS, STILL JOINED,
ARE RAISED IT IS *PARAVARTITA* (TURNING).

IF WITHIN THE CAVE OF HER THIGHS
YOU SIT ROTATING YOUR HIPS LIKE A BLACK BEE,
IT IS *MARKATA* (THE MONKEY).

AND IF, IN THIS POSE, YOU TURN AWAY FROM HER,
IT IS *MARDITAKA* (CRUSHING SPICES).

SHE SITS WITH RAISED THIGHS,
HER FEET PLACED EITHER SIDE OF YOUR WAIST;
LINGA ENTERS YONI; YOU RAIN HARD BLOWS UPON HER BODY:
THIS IS *KSHUDGAGA* (STRIKING).

SEATED ERECT, THE LOVELY GIRL FOLDS ONE LEG TO HER BODY
AND STRETCHES THE OTHER ALONG THE BED, WHILE YOU MIRROR HER ACTIONS:
THIS IS *YUGMAPADA* (THE FEET YOKE).

IF, WITH LEFT LEG EXTENDED,
SHE ENCIRCLES YOUR WAIST WITH HER RIGHT LEG,
LAYING ITS ANKLE ACROSS HER LEFT THIGH,
AND YOU DO THE SAME,
IT IS *Swastika* (THE SWASTIKA)*.

SITTING FACE TO FACE IN BED,
HER BREASTS PRESSED TIGHT AGAINST YOUR CHEST,
LET EACH OF YOU LOCK HEELS
BEHIND THE OTHER'S WAIST,
AND LEAN BACK CLASPING ONE ANOTHER'S WRISTS.
NOW, SET THE SWING GENTLY IN MOTION,
YOUR BELOVED, IN PRETENDED FEAR,
CLINGING TO YOUR BODY WITH HER FLAWLESS LIMBS,
COOING AND MOANING WITH PLEASURE:
THIS IS *Dolita* (THE SWING).

SEATED, THE LADY RAISES
ONE FOOT TO POINT VERTICALLY OVER HER HEAD
AND STEADIES IT WITH HER HANDS,
OFFERING UP HER YONI FOR LOVEMAKING:
THIS IS *Mayura* (THE PEACOCK).

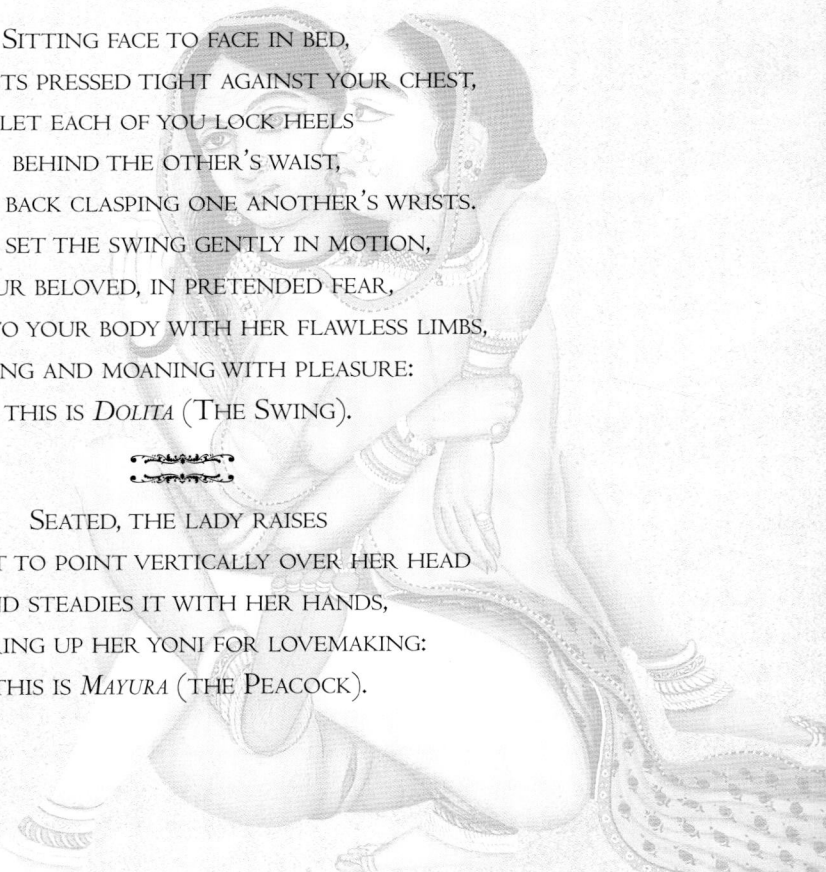

If, sitting facing her,
you grasp her ankles and fasten them like a chain
behind your neck, and she
grips her toes as you make love,
it is the delightful *Padma* (the Lotus).

Sitting erect, grip your lover's waist
and pull her on to you,
your loins continuously leaping together
with a sound like the flapping of elephants' ears:
this is *Kirtibandha* (the Knot of Fame).

Kneeling between her thighs,
tickle her breasts and under her arms,
call her 'my lovely darling'
and print deep nail marks around her nipples:
thus *Jaya* (Victory) is expounded.

Standing positions

Couples who make love standing are very frequently depicted on the walls of temples such as Khajuraho and Konarak. Making love against a support of a wall of a pillar is known as *Sthita* or steadying:

WHEN THE WOMAN SITS IN HER LOVER'S
CRADLED HANDS, HER ARMS AROUND HIS NECK,
THIGHS GRIPPING HIS WAIST,
HER FEET PUSHING BACK AND FORTH AGAINST A WALL,
IT IS *AVALAMBITAKA* (SUSPENDED).

WHEN, CATCHING AND CRUSHING YOUR LOVER IN THE CAGE OF YOUR ARMS,
YOU FORCE HER KNEES APART WITH YOURS AND SINK SLOWLY INTO HER,
IT IS *DADHYAYATAKA* (CHURNING CURDS).

WHEN SHE LEANS AGAINST A WALL,
PLANTING HER FEET AS WIDELY APART AS POSSIBLE, AND YOU ENTER THE CAVE
BETWEEN HER THIGHS, EAGER FOR LOVEMAKING,
IT IS *SAMMUKHA* (FACE-TO-FACE).

IF, AS YOU LEAN AGAINST THE WALL,
YOUR LADY TWINES HER THIGHS AROUND YOURS,
LOCKS HER FEET TO YOUR KNEES, AND CLASPS YOUR NECK, MAKING LOVE
VERY PASSIONATELY, IT IS *DOLA* (THE SWING).

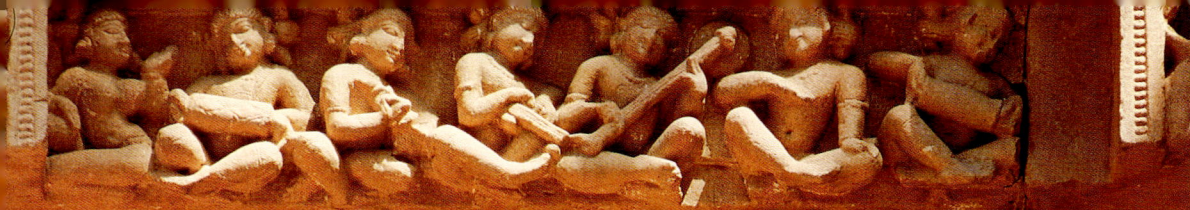

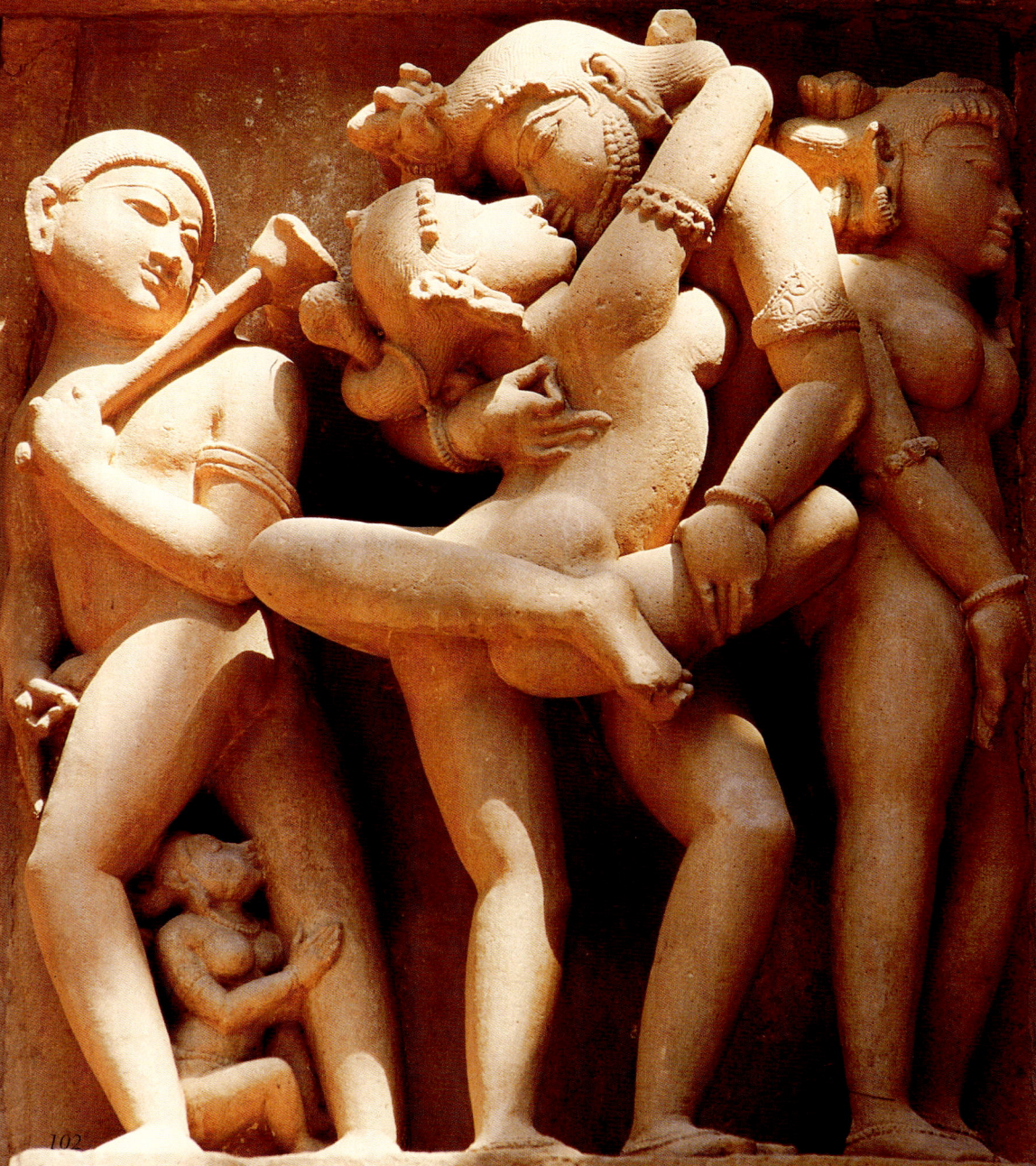

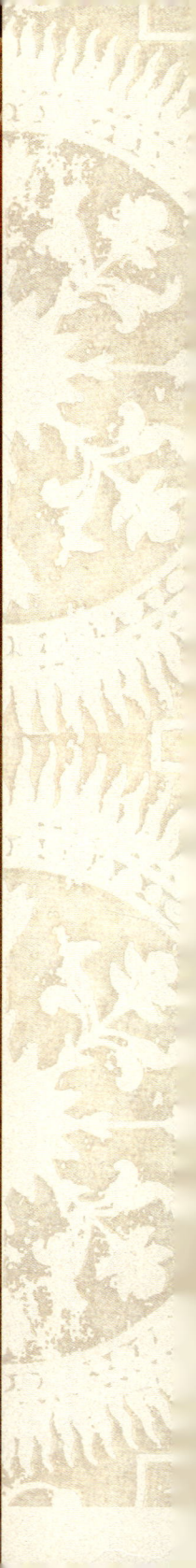

When your lover draws up one leg,
allowing the heel to nestle just behind your knee,
and you make love, embracing her forcefully,
it is *Traivikrama* (the Stride).

If you catch one of her knees
firmly in your hand and stand making love with her
while her hands explore and caress your body,
it is *Tripadam* (the Tripod).

If she raises one leg and you catch hold of her little foot,
caressing her breasts and telling her how much you love her,
it is *Ekapada* (One Foot).

Her foot pressed to your heart,
your arms encircling and supporting her,
lean back against the wall and enjoy the lovely girl:
this is *Veshta* (the Encircling).

She stands against the wall, lotus-hands on hips,
long, lovely fingers reaching to her navel.
Cup her foot in your palm and let your free hand caress her limbs.
Put your arm around her neck
and enjoy her as she leans there at her ease.
Vatsyayana and others who knew the art of love in its great days
called this posture *Tala* (the Palm).

Oral Pleasures

Ancient Sanskrit medical texts identify oral sex as a defining homosexual act as well as with masculinity in women. Even in the *Kama Sutra* oral sex techniques are prescribed though not recommended by Vatsyayana who expresses no moral outrage at the sexual desires of people of the 'third nature'. Saying that oral sex is not wrong for one who frequents courtesans and if it is a 'custom of the country or region', he describes oral sex as an act between 'two kinds of eunuchs, who are disguised either as males, or as females. The acts that are done on the *jaghana* or middle parts of women, are done in the mouths by these eunuchs, and this is called *auparishtaka*.'

Although the text says that *auparishtaka* is practised only by unchaste and wanton women, female attendants and serving maids, that is, those who are not married to anybody, and those 'who live by shampooing', it recognizes that 'male servants of some men carry on mouth congress with their masters and that it is also practised by some citizens, who know each other well.' Almost extolling the pleasures of oral sex he adds: 'For the sake of such things courtesans abandon men possessed of good qualities, liberal and clever, and become attached to low persons, such as slaves and elephant drivers (who perform oral sex).' He adds that oral sex can be a stimulant and can arouse men who, due to age or other excesses, have trouble getting an erection.

Acknowledged to be extremely arousing, both cunnilingus and fellatio are more than purely tactile activities as they involve other physical and emotional elements. They are the highest expressions of love that can be exchanged between two people, and because they involve the primary sex organs, the experience can be intense. Men love the sensation of their penis deep inside the other's throat as there are so many more nerve endings at the tip of the penis, and using the lips to move up and down the phallus can be the surest route to orgasm. Besides the penis there are other parts

Facing page: Decorating or pelting each another with flowers from the Kadamba tree is known as udakakashvedika *or sporting in the water.*

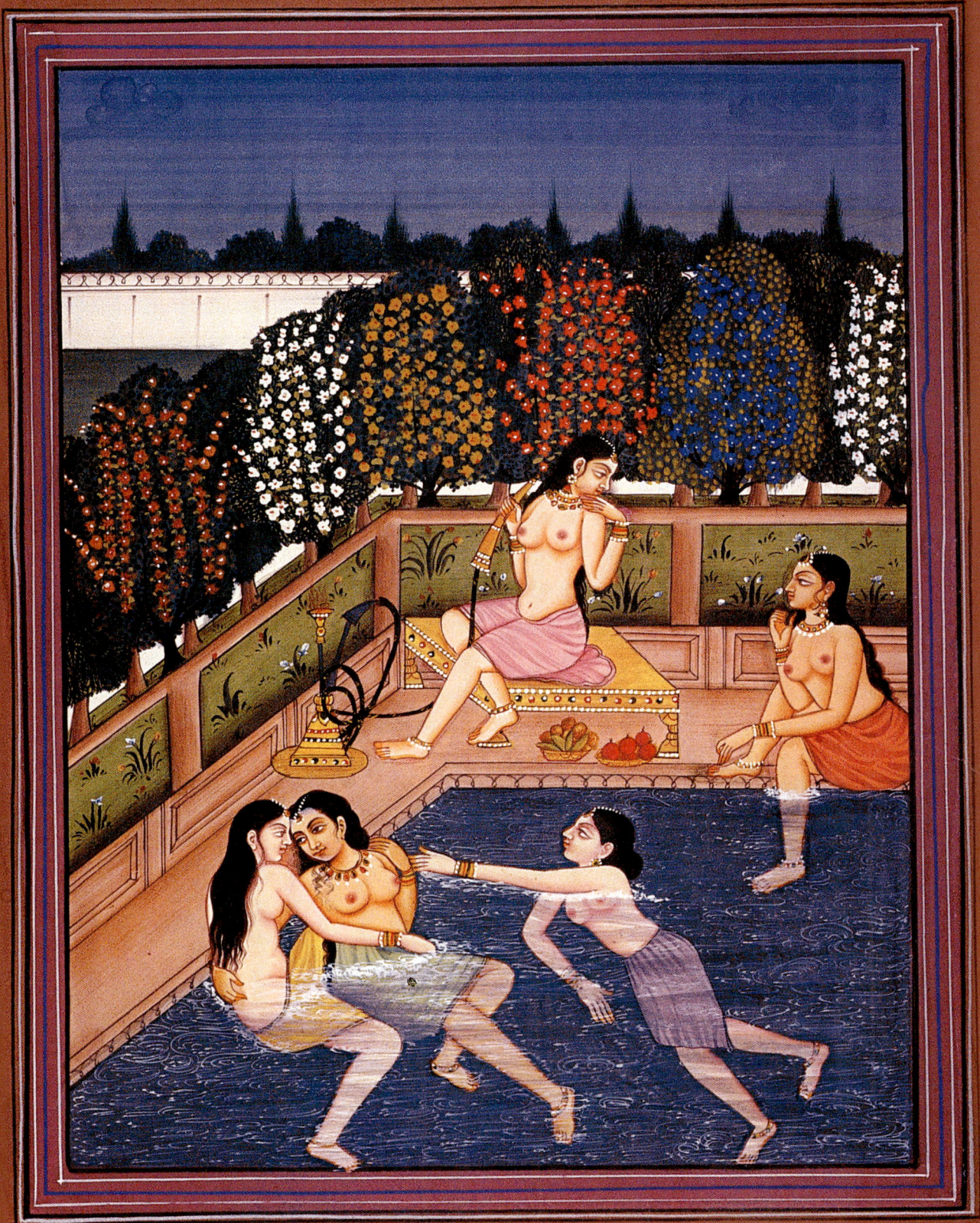

of a man's body: men are particularly sensitive around the nipples that respond just as well to oral stimulation.

The same is equally true of women. Cunnilingus is a form of oral sex involving mouth contact with the vagina and is derived from two Latin words: *cunnus* or the vulva, and *lingere* or licking. In cunnilingus, the labia, the clitoris and the vaginal area are licked, kissed or gently sucked. Since for lesbians foreplay and oral sex makes up for most part of the sexual experience, cunnilingus plays an exceedingly important role as a number of women are known to immediately experience orgasm by, 'placing the tip of the tongue just outside the vagina, the woman kisses and licks the lady's temple of love. And with the lips sucks her fluids'. Ancient as well as medieval texts talk about and describe in detail the G-spot. Named after its discoverer, Dr. Ernst Grafenberg, the G-spot is defined as a flat area about the size of a coin, two inches deep inside the vagina. It's just behind the pubic bone, on the vaginal wall that is closest to the belly button and can be reached with the index finger. The *Pururavasamanasijasutra*, a 12th-century text describes its equivalent called a *sardagrdi* as a place which is like a lily inside a woman's vagina located four fingers deep right behind the navel. The other amazingly modern idea expressed in this text is that not only do women have sexual desires but they have 'eight times the capability of men to have orgasms'. Vatsyayana also recognized that women often perform oral sex on one another. 'Some women of the harem, when they are amorous, do the acts of the mouth on the *yonis* of one another, and some men do the same thing with women. The way of doing this (that is, of kissing the *yoni*) should be known to be different from kissing the mouth.'

The *Kama Sutra* then goes on to describe various techniques of oral sex. While none of the postures or techniques is exclusively the preserve of either heterosexual or homosexual couples, they can easily be adapted or modified to suit one's sexual proclivities. There are eight oral techniques that the *Kama Sutra* says 'are done by people of the third sex one after the other'. These include cunnilingus techniques like:

WITH DELICATE FINGERTIPS,
PINCH THE ARCHED LIPS OF HER HOUSE OF LOVE
VERY VERY SLOWLY TOGETHER,
AND KISS THEM AS THOUGH YOU KISSED HER LOWER LIP:
THIS IS *ADHARA-SPHURITAM* (THE QUIVERING KISS).

NOW SPREAD, INDEED CLEAVE ASUNDER,
THAT ARCHWAY WITH YOUR NOSE AND LET YOUR TONGUE
GENTLY PROBE HER *YONI* (VAGINA),
WITH YOUR NOSE, LIPS AND CHIN SLOWLY CIRCLING:
IT BECOMES *JIHVA-BHRAMANAKA* (THE CIRCLING TONGUE).

LET YOUR TONGUE REST FOR A MOMENT
IN THE ARCHWAY TO THE FLOWER-BOWED LORD'S TEMPLE
BEFORE ENTERING TO WORSHIP VIGOROUSLY,
CAUSING HER SEED TO FLOW:
THIS IS *JIHVA-MARDITA* (THE TONGUE MASSAGE).

NEXT, FASTEN YOUR LIPS TO HERS
AND TAKE DEEP KISSES
FROM THIS LOVELY ONE, YOUR BELOVED,
NIBBLING AT HER AND SUCKING HARD AT HER CLITORIS:
THIS IS CALLED *CHUSHITA* (SUCKED).

Cup, lift her young buttocks,
let your tongue-tip probe her navel, slither down
to rotate skillfully in the archway
of the love-god's dwelling and lap her love-water:
this is *Uchchushita* (Sucked Up).

Stirring the root of her thighs,
which her own hands
are gripping and holding widely apart,
your fluted tongue drinks at her sacred spring:
this is *Kshobhaka* (Stirring).

Place your darling on a couch,
set her feet to your shoulders, clasp her waist,
suck hard and let your tongue stir
her overflowing love-temple:
this is called *Bahuchushita* (Sucked Hard).

If the pair of you lie side by side,
facing opposite ways,
and kiss each other's secret parts
using the techniques described above,
it is known as *Kakila* (the Crow).

(From Indra Sinha's *Kama Sutra*)

Besides cunnilingus, the *Kama Sutra* also describes fellatio techniques as even heterosexual men like oral sex, described in the *Kama Sutra* as techniques usually adopted by people of the third sex. The text does not encourage oral sex, but some of the techniques include:

When, holding the man's *lingam* with his hand, and placing it between his lips, the eunuch moves about his mouth, it is called the `nominal congress'. This first step is called also called *Nimitta* (Touching).

When, covering the end of the *lingam* with his fingers collected together like the bud of a plant or flower, the eunuch presses the sides of it with his lips, using his teeth also, it is called *Parshvatoddashta* (Biting the sides).

When, being desired to proceed, the eunuch presses the end of the *lingam* with his lips closed together, and kisses it as if he were drawing it out, it is called the *Bahiha-samdansha* or the Outer Pincers.

When being asked to go on, he puts the *lingam* further into his mouth, and presses it with his lips and then takes it out, it is called the *Antaha-samdansha* or the Inner Pincers.

When, holding the *lingam* in his hand, the eunuch kisses it as if he were kissing the lower lip, it is called Kissing or *Chumbitaka*.

When, after kissing it, he touches it with his tongue everywhere, and passes the tongue over the end of it, it is called *Parimrshtaka* or Rubbing.

The use of artificial penises or dildos were also known and described in detail. 'Generally, union with a rectilinear object *(riju)* is termed as normal copulation.' The text goes on to describe women in harems who penetrate one another with vegetables. In yet another medieval text called the *Manmata Samhita*, a paean to the God of Love, there is a detailed description of how to make, and use a dildo. In the *Kama Sutra* several postures known variously as 'the devastator', 'the cruel', and 'the thunderbolt', involve using force when inserting and vibrating the dildo.

There is no one proper or correct way to perform oral sex. Specific skills, techniques, and positions are not as important as one's own desire to please and be pleasured. There are two people involved, with their own needs and desires. Oral sex, like all human acts, has to be learned, and learning anything takes time and patience.

Adhorata—ANAL SEX

In order for lovers to expand their sexual repertoire and explore all avenues of pleasure, the *Kama Sutra* makes note of the fact that certain people from the southern part of India resort to anal sex. While the rear entry intercourse that is referred to by Vatsyayana is for heterosexual couples, anal sex is also the preferred course of sexual behaviour for homosexual men and thus easily adapted to suit their needs. While the *Manusmriti* admonishes sexual intercourse among ordinary males (*pums-prakrti*), the atonement is a mere ritual bathing and applies only to brahmanas: 'A twice-born man who engages in intercourse with a male, or with a female in a cart drawn by oxen, in water, or in the daytime, shall bathe, dressed in his clothes.' (*Manusmriti* 11.175)

So, anal eroticism, was and may well still be surrounded by taboo, although millions of men and women—straight, gay or bisexual continue to experiment with it. The *Kama Sutra* acknowledged what Kinsey stated thirty-five years ago: that the anal region had erotic significance for a large part of the population worldwide.

There are several forms of anal sex. The least practised, contrary to common belief, is anal penetration because touching, stroking and masturbating are more common. Some people enjoy the sensation of a finger on their own or a lover's anal opening, others prefer the insertion of a dildo and still others seek complete penetration to achieve an orgasm. Like the vagina, there is a very high concentration of nerve endings in and around the anal opening itself. Hence any stimulation in the region is immediately pleasurable. The prostate which is immediately behind the rectal wall can be a source of pleasure when massaged by a finger, a dildo or a penis. Anal pleasure can be psychological as well as physical, for the associated taboo adds to the thrill of experiencing the forbidden, while sharing it with a partner is an act of openness and giving.

The sexual positions that a couple prefer depend on a variety of factors like physical comfort, who is the more dominant partner, preferences, inhibitions. Sometimes the capacity to prolong or hasten orgasms too determines sexual positions. Known to be exceedingly pleasurable, this form of intercourse allows for deep penetration and vigorous pushing if the couple wants it.

Ancient sages believed that humans could learn a lot about lovemaking from animals. They advised lovers to study the mating patterns of certain animals, which is how the rear entry position has become a classic position. For women, the same can be done by using a dildo. For lesbians, the active partner, the woman behind can don an artificial penis and penetrate her partner vaginally. Gentle massage around and slowly inside the rectum can unleash powerful sources of untapped sexual energy and life force. The following are rear entry positions that are again easy to adapt:

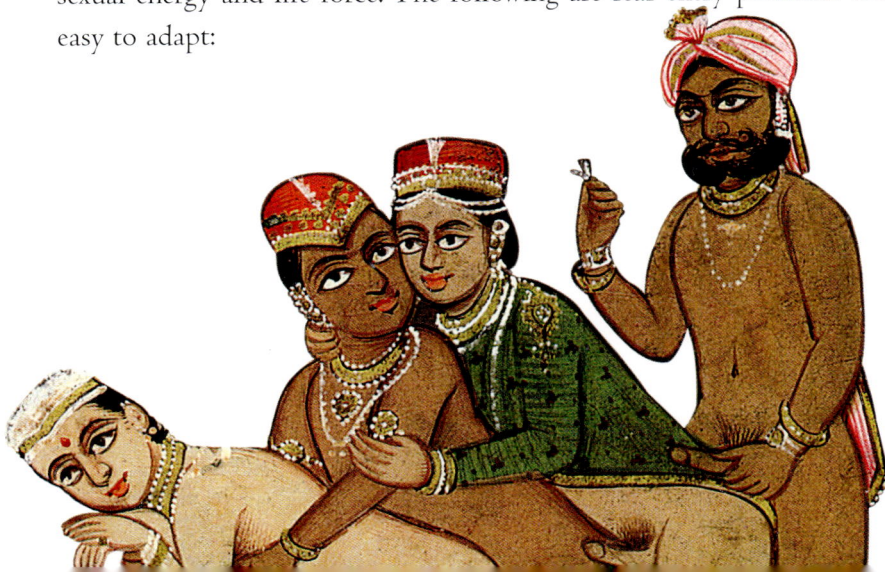

IF YOU MOUNT HIM LIKE A DOG, GRIPPING HIS WAIST,

AND HE TWISTS ROUND TO GAZE INTO YOUR FACE,

EXPERTS IN THE ART OF LOVE SAY IT IS *SVANAKA* (THE DOG).

SHE BENDS WELL FORWARD AND GRIPS

THE BEDSTEAD, HER BUTTOCKS RAISED HIGH;

CUP YOUR HANDS TO SERPENTS' HOODS

AND SQUEEZE HER JAR-SHAPED BREASTS TOGETHER:

THIS IS *DHENUKA* (THE MILCH COW).

IF A LADY, EAGER FOR LOVE,

GOES ON ALL FOURS, HUMPING HER BACK LIKE A DOE,

AND YOU ENJOY HER FROM BEHIND,

RUTTING AS THOUGH YOU'D LOST ALL HUMAN NATURE,

IT IS *HIRANA* (THE DEER).

WHEN, WITH LOTUS-FEET SET WELL APART ON THE GROUND, HE BENDS,

PLACING A HAND UPON EACH THIGH, AND YOU TAKE HIM FROM THE REAR,

IT IS *GARDABHA* (THE ASS).

SHE LIES ON HER FRONT, GRASPING HER ANKLES IN HER OWN HANDS

AND PULLING THEM UP BEHIND HER:

THIS DIFFICULT POSTURE IS KNOWN TO EXPERTS

AS *MALLAKA* (THE WRESTLER).

LYING ON HIS SIDE, FACING AWAY,
THE FAWN-EYED YOUNG MAN
OFFERS YOU HIS BUTTOCKS
AND YOUR PENIS PENETRATES THE HOUSE OF LOVE:
THIS IS *NAGABANDHA* (THE SERPENT).

YOU LIFT HER ANKLES HIGH;
SHE DRAWS UP
AND EXTENDS HER LEGS AS THOUGH SHE WERE
CRAWLING THROUGH THE AIR:
THIS IS *HASTIKA* (THE ELEPHANT).

SHE STANDS ON HER PALMS AND FEET;
YOU STAND BEHIND HER
AND LIFT ONE OF HER FEET TO YOUR SHOULDER,
ENJOYING THE LOVELY GIRL:
THIS IS *TRAIVIKRAMA* (THE STRIDE).

SEIZE HER FEET AND LIFT THEM HIGH
(LIKE A WHEEL BARROW),
DRIVE YOUR PENIS INTO HER *YONI*
AND PLEASURE HER WITH VIGOROUS STROKES:
THIS IS *KULISHA* (THE THUNDERBOLT).

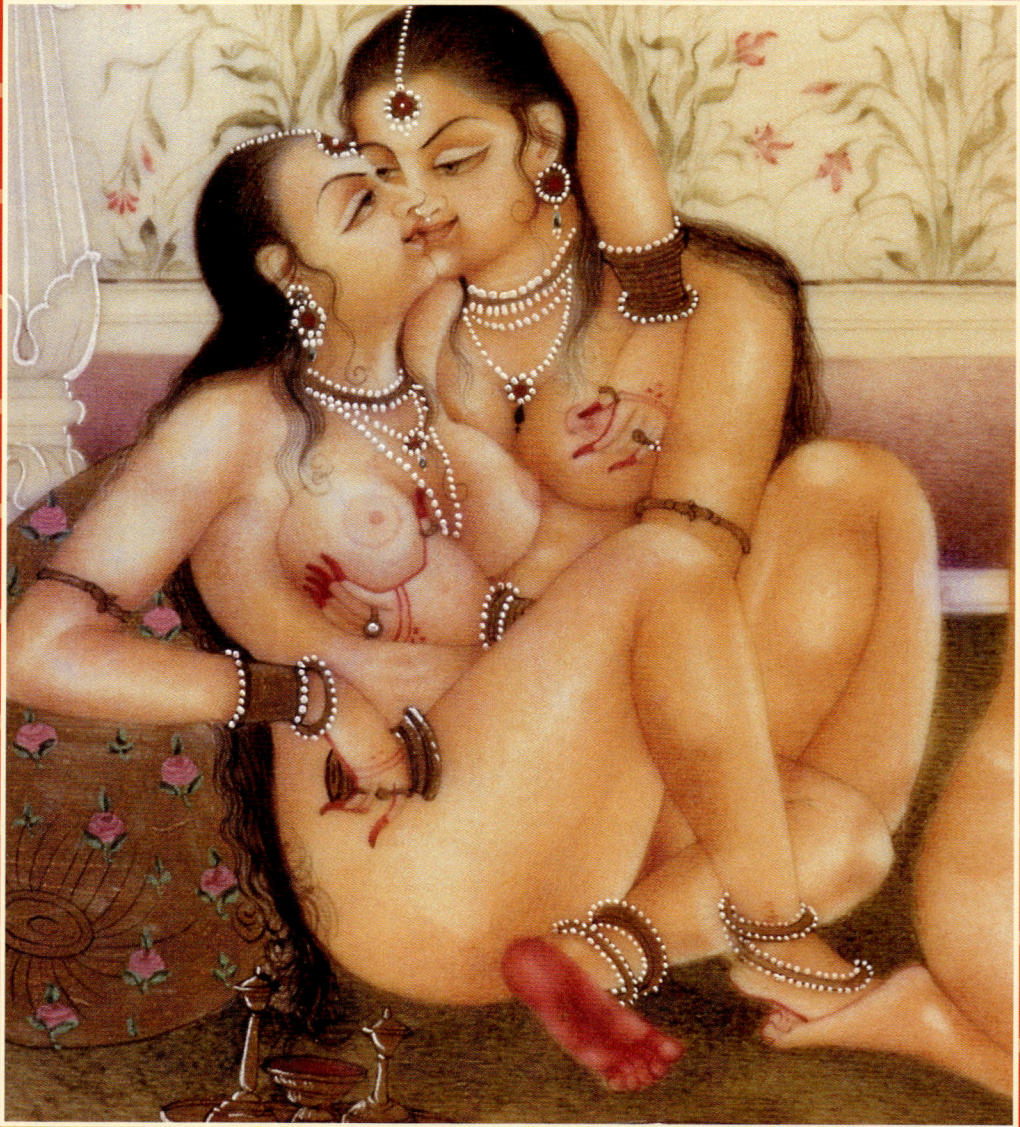

Conclusion

Society in the 21st century considers itself to be advanced and expansive in thought and deed but continues to grapple with age-old issues. Dichotomies that revolve around the concepts of war and peace, commerce and culture, spirituality and sexuality remain unchanged and unresolved as controversies about the basic needs of what human beings want remain unaddressed through the centuries. Modern life demands reconciling diverse opinions, situations and mindsets and finding a middle path for a balanced existence. For freedom is a tenuous mistress often making more demands than the more comfortable boundaries within which civilizations have thus far flourished. Threatened by a world that is changing too rapidly for comprehension, where clearly demarcated ideals of right and wrong are

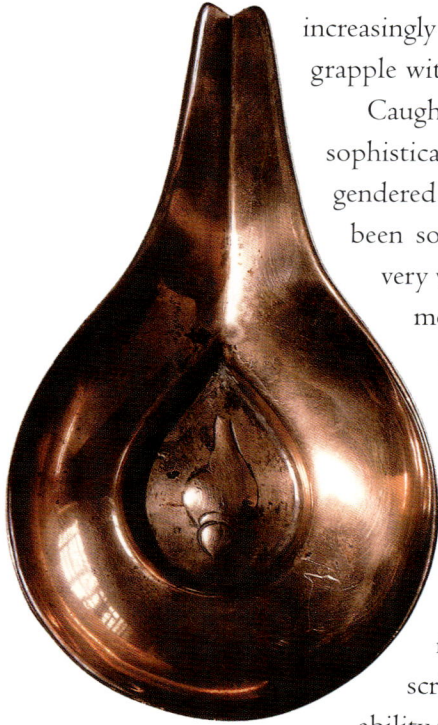

increasingly turning out to be only shades of gray, human beings grapple with moral fluidity.

Caught in the quagmire even as people purport to grow more sophisticated is the position and rights of gay and other third-gendered groups. Over the past three decades sexual identity has been so debated, alternatively maligned and glorified, that the very word begs redefining today. Just what does sexual identity mean? Some see it as a defining gender, others as being the object of one's affections either from the opposite or same sex; some say that homosexuality, heterosexuality and bisexuality have always existed across history and cultures and reflect an essential aspect of human experience; still others see sexuality as a byproduct of historical and cultural understanding based on social definitions and thus not an inherent part of an individual. Even evolved traditions like the Hindu scriptures have traditionally based sexual identity on the ability to procreate. While it accepted physical attraction for the same sex because it abounds in nature, social parameters were formed to preserve the rights of progeny, especially those of sons. Modern societies, however, clearly recognize that human relationships have so many more dimensions to them than merely passing on genetic material, and thereby debunk the myth that sexuality is only for procreation. 'Human worth is not to be measured only in terms of fertility,' society seems to declare.

The exact definition of sexual identify may still be open to debate but general attitudes towards homosexuality seem to be better defined. Even as sexual preferences come to the fore and find expression, the rest of society wrestles with myths that refuse to go away. Gay people are oftentimes shunned and rejected as

Modern societies recognize that relationships have so many more dimensions to them and thereby debunk the myth that sexuality is only for procreation.

being immoral and undeserving of any rights based solely on their sexual proclivities. Homosexuals are considered to be a threat to society. Should they be feared? Are they a harmful, corruptive force? Society continues to believe that homosexuals sexually abuse children, that you can `spot' a gay person by his mannerisms, that homosexuality is an illness—a result of psychological problems, the list runs on. But the most important misconception that people harbour is that gays are promiscuous, have multiple partners and are unable to form or stay in long-term relationships. Given all these problems would denying them their basic rights and privileges help? Or should society be progressive enough to accept as 'simply another colour within the rainbow of human variety'.

In the earlier stages of civilization, family structures remained undefined groups living together in loose groupings; paternity did not matter as long as the children were looked after by the community. With the discovery of the male role in reproduction, however, and the rise of patriarchy, the stage was set for the emergence of sexual identities. As worship of the womb turned into reverence for semen the mother goddess cults made way for phallus worship. In many early cultures, there were initiation rituals in which young men became adults by being inseminated by older men; 'maleness' had to be passed on and sex between males was the process by which masculinity was acquired. Within some of these communities, homosexual activity was essential rather than a threat to masculinity.

Subsequent urbanization, industrialization and economic growth meant that those who were ambiguous about their sexuality could leave behind their families and seek a personal life. Cities allowed groups of people who felt differently to come together in relative anonymity, and develop alternative lifestyles. At first, these

The worship of the womb made way for reverence for semen
further paving the path for phallus worship.

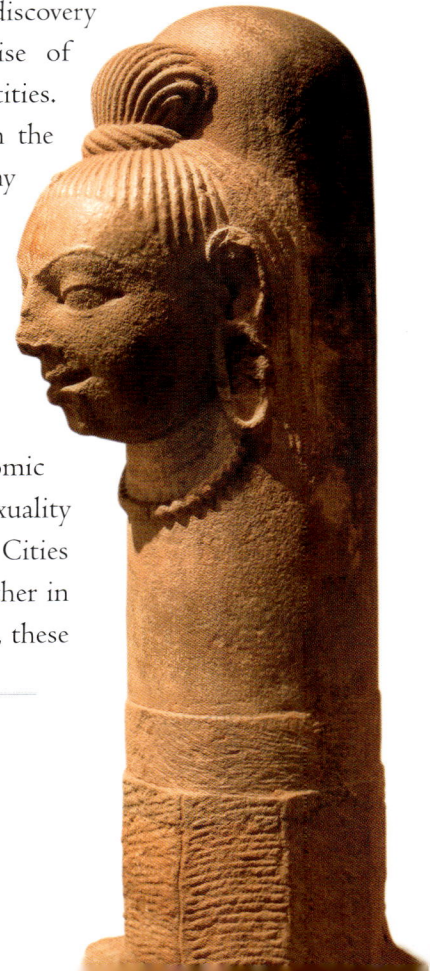

groups were secretive and subjected to strong persecution. During the 20th century, however, this gave way to even more complex social networks and to a sense of community among self-identified homosexuals, who were beginning to resist the manner in which they were being labelled as sick and inadequate. In 1948 Dr Alfred C Kinsey's report ended these speculations and deconstructed accepted prototypes of sexual orientation. This was the basis for the gay liberation movement which reclaimed equal validity of homosexuality with heterosexuality; rejected medical terms, and popularized new descriptions, such as 'gay', emphasized the importance of 'coming out', being identified as a lesbian or a gay man; and, above all, it affirmed the importance of taking pride in being lesbian and gay.

The strength of these new identities, however, soon came under fire with the emergence of AIDS, and while it had the effect of producing a new solidarity among lesbians and gay men, the need for safe sex and monogamous relationships became important. Uncanny as it may seem, ancient Indian scriptures and even treatises like the *Kama Sutra* preach that one's orientation or preferences notwithstanding, it was important to express one's sexual nature responsibly; they taught a lesson not of hedonism but of restraint and moral sexuality. Although widely viewed as a treatise that describes impossible techniques and sexual positions, the *Kama Sutra* actually provides a window to an extremely sophisticated Hindu heritage, very different from the one conveyed in most philosophical, historical and religious discourses. It considers promiscuous behaviour, heterosexual or homosexual, as a problem for the emotional and spiritual well-being of individuals and endeavours to inculcate correct and responsible conduct in all human beings, a lesson that now appears to have been lost. Today, sex is as much about instant gratification and seeking one's pleasure wherever whenever available than about attentiveness and responsible behaviour. What appears to be lacking, despite the efforts of governments and societies, is knowledge. For instance, can HIV and other STDs be sexually transmitted by lesbians during sex? Most lesbians don't think so; actually fluids such as vaginal secretions and menstrual blood are considered much more high risk because these facilitate virus transmission. It is equally high risk to have these fluids come into contact with broken skin or thin membranes, such as the anal lining. So, nibbling that does not break the skin, is erotic and fun as is sucking on the ears and neck which are wonderfully safe. Other questions that are often asked are: How safe is oral sex? How important is it to ensure that while rimming your partner the area be covered with either a latex or dental dam? Oral sex is indeed low risk, but there is increased risk if the woman has cuts or sores on her mouth, or her partner receiving oral sex has sores on her genitals or is having her periods. Sharing sex toys and vibrators can also be risky if they have vaginal fluids, blood or faeces on them.

Hygiene being a major concern, before you even consider doing anything make certain that your partner is clean. Hindus have always believed that cleanliness is next only to godliness and this becomes almost imperative when it comes to intercourse between same-sex partners. Hygiene, for example, should always be the first priority in any act of anal penetration. A condom on a finger inserted into the anus can aid lubrication as well as protect against scratches. Wash and cleanse thoroughly before and after anal sex. Almost anticipating the problems of AIDS and other sexually transmitted diseases, treatises like the *Kama Sutra* place a great deal of emphasis on personal hygiene as well as the need to pay attention to one's own appearance and surroundings. It advises men on the art of seduction, on how to go about setting the right environment and pace. First and foremost, it advises one to take a bath, a long luxurious one using scented perfumes, to clip one's nails, and that the hair be well cut, groomed and pomaded. It then advises cleaning up the room and setting the mood, beds that have clean silk sheets, music playing in the background, scented candles and incense sticks, jasmine flowers and rose petals, and paintings on the wall. There should be no place for anything that is ugly, malodorous, or shabby when it comes to the act of making love. Thus beyond satisfying one's lust and longings, the *Kama Sutra* is really about mastering these desires. Truly good lovers are ones who develop a heightened awareness of, and control over all of their senses, and are rooted in the present that impacts one's whole life.

While it has become necessary to address sexual issues especially those like AIDS, a vast section of modern society continues to shy away from discussing third-sex issues, preferring to hide behind the shield of morality and religion;

religious institutions too are unable to come to a consensus on homosexuality. Society indeed does not see gay people as being spiritually adept and are by and large of the opinion that the gay movement runs contrary to prevailing religious beliefs and is hence rejected by most religious denominations. But despite one's choice of sexual partners, same-sex people too have a right to seek fulfilment both sexual and spiritual, and seek a proper place in society. But how can one reconcile homosexuality with spirituality?

Gender differences are part of the diversity of created forms, and tradition teaches us that such diversity can only be harmonized, not by homogenizing, opposing or denying forms, but by accepting them and transcending them. Ancient India has always believed that the force of sex is one way or path to seek the highest spiritual energy; and this can be done neither by confining sexuality within an arbitrary social order, nor by renouncing it, but by total submission to it. The cosmic energy stored in human sexuality was indeed revered and worshipped in India as the primal force and called *Shakti* or power. There is a very close connection between sexuality and spirituality in both the Hindu philosophy and Tantra with Indian scriptures like the *Upanishads* considering the human body with all its innate attributes, physical and psychological, as sacred.

Moreover, according to Indian philosophy, it is only after acquiring thorough knowledge about an experience that one can be in a position to transcend it; that the three basic purposes of human life—to live a righteous life, to acquire wealth, to experience the pleasures of sex and parenthood, have to be first served, if they have to be renounced. This, among other things, was an acknowledgment of the fact that the higher the awareness of the sacredness of the physical, the more heightened will be the sexual pleasure. Sexuality thus seen as a pathway to bliss was a means of experiencing the Divine, a way thereby of sublimating the sexual experience to a higher purpose. Carl Jung himself linked homoeroticism to sacred experiences: '...he is endowed with a wealth of religious feelings...and a spiritual

Facing page: In Tantra, sexual energy was seen as a primal force and became synonymous with Shakti worship.

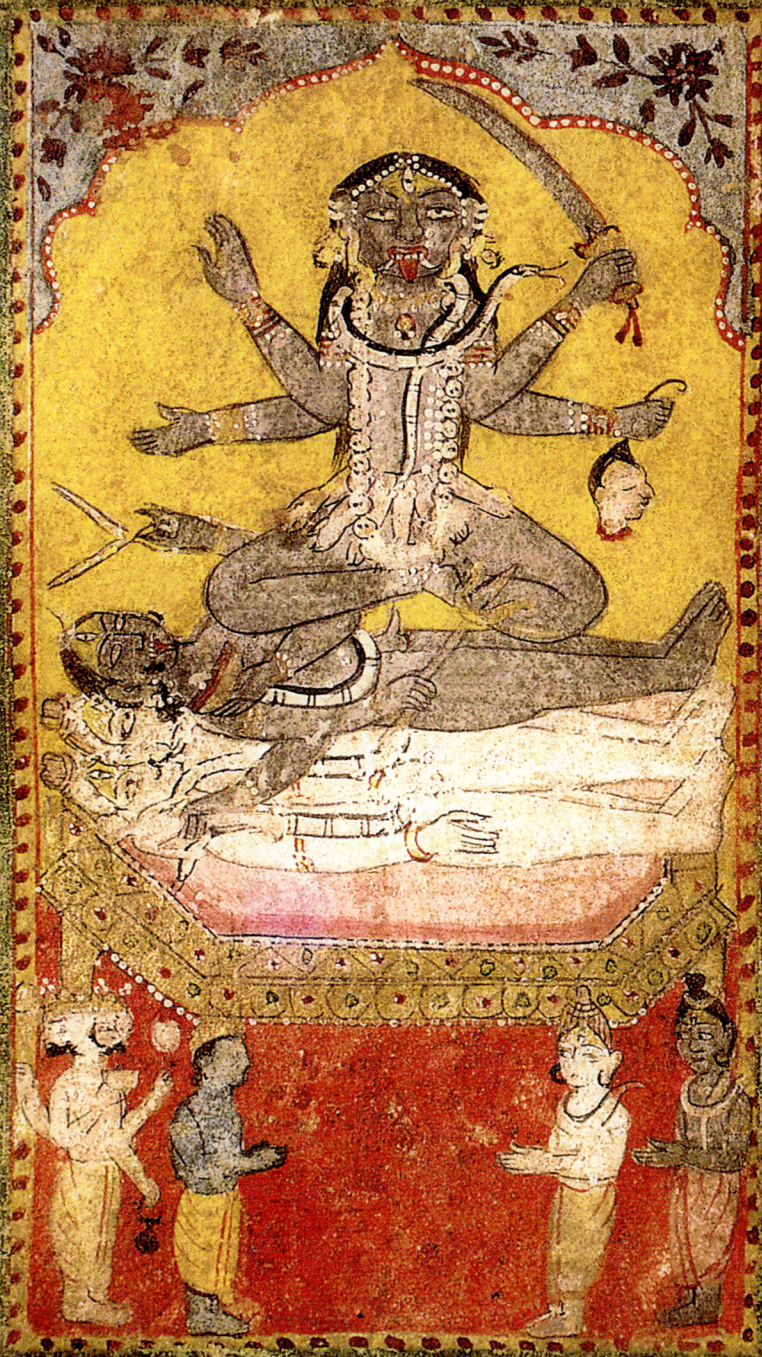

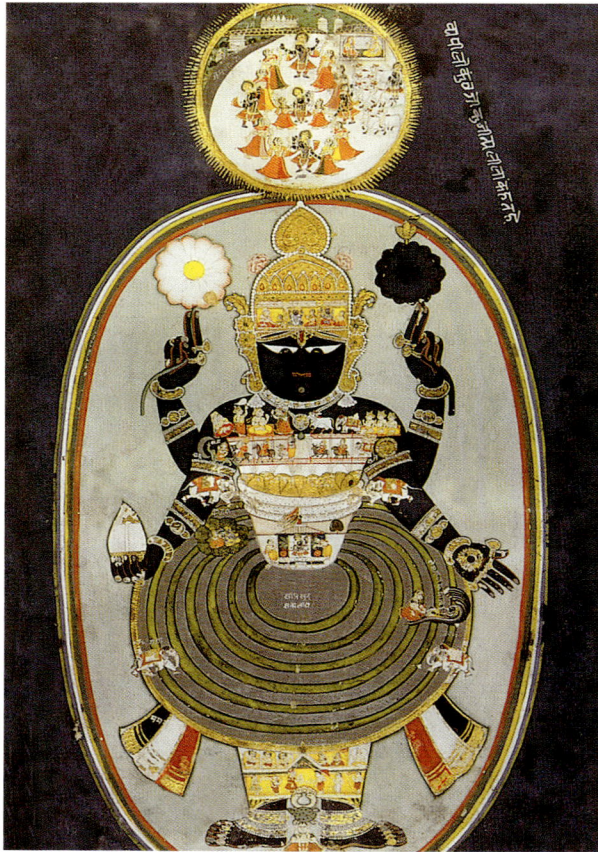

receptivity which makes him responsive to revelation,' he wrote in 1980. Sublimation in some cases may take the form of chastity or even androgynous unity. But sublimation does not necessarily require sexual abstinence, rather a lesson in how not to become a slave to one's passions and tap into the full power that lies within them. Tradition also teaches us that reality is *Satyam, Shivam Sunderam* that is the harmonious combination of all that it True, Good and Beautiful. The scriptures excluded no one from engaging in spiritual practices because of class, character, social standing, gender, race.

Sexuality was seen as a pathway to bliss, a means of experiencing the divine.

122

Given that everything is God's creation, one has to learn to respect diversity in all its forms, accepting it as God's *lila* or interplay in the universe. Accepting homosexuals in society is one way of accepting the diversity of life. For ultimately the gay movement is about human dignity, individual rights and values, the discovery of new potentials for the self, and above all, about love. These are the higher values that not just gay people but all human beings should strive for.

Modern conceptions of free love and sexual hedonism are a parody of these basic principles. Contemporary society tends to accept only that which is a scientific and technical truth, which is factual and objective, ignoring the mystical and spiritual realms of life. Understanding one's sexuality and coming to terms with it are becoming imperative today, but the need of the hour is to go with the flow. And certainly society is doing just that. Cultural norms are changing as is amply demonstrated by the media, popular culture and public attitudes. Even two decades ago, homosexuality would have been a frightening realization but today young people are exploring all their options before settling on an identity. And more and more people are inventing their own labels, and not just sexual, rather than having any imposed on them by the world. The new awareness and openness has brought gays together as a people and allowed them to examine their lives, for sexual flexibility is not about rebellion, it is about freedom of choice. It is for both heterosexuals and homosexuals to understand that rather than rebelling against nature, accepting one's destiny is the true mark of a mature society. Amara Dasa says it best in his book *The Third Gender:* 'It is important that we appreciate a world filled with variety. There will never be just one race, one gender, one colour, one sound, or one anything. The Vedas describe this material world as a reflection of an infinitely beautiful, perfect, and eternal spiritual world that has even more variety than we can imagine. We are all a part of this variegatedness, and we all have our own unique role to play. It is therefore pointless to argue over who is higher, lower, more important, less important, etc. We all have our own individual, intrinsic nature, and part of that nature is that we all serve God. That loving mood is eternal and full of unlimited bliss.'

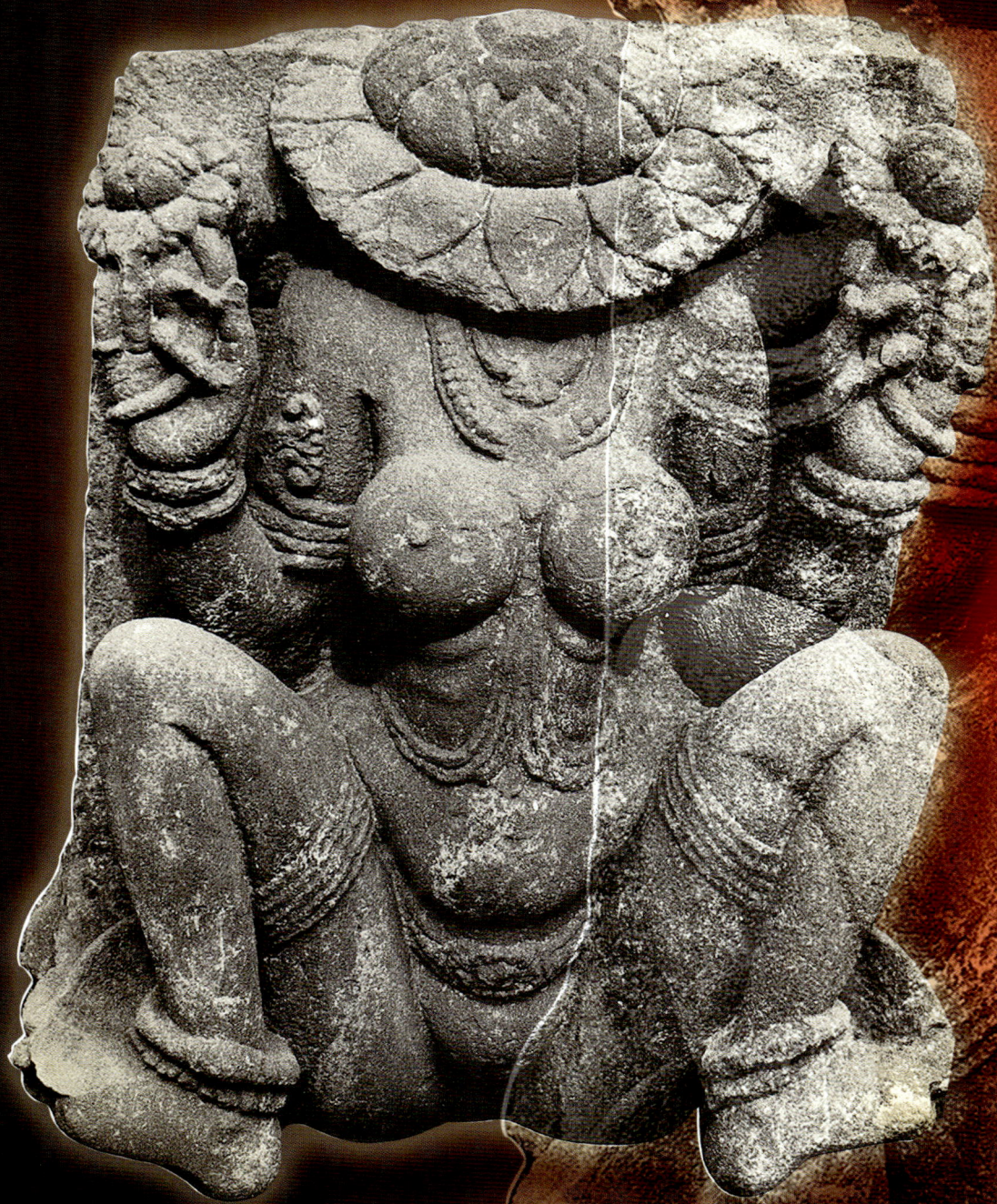

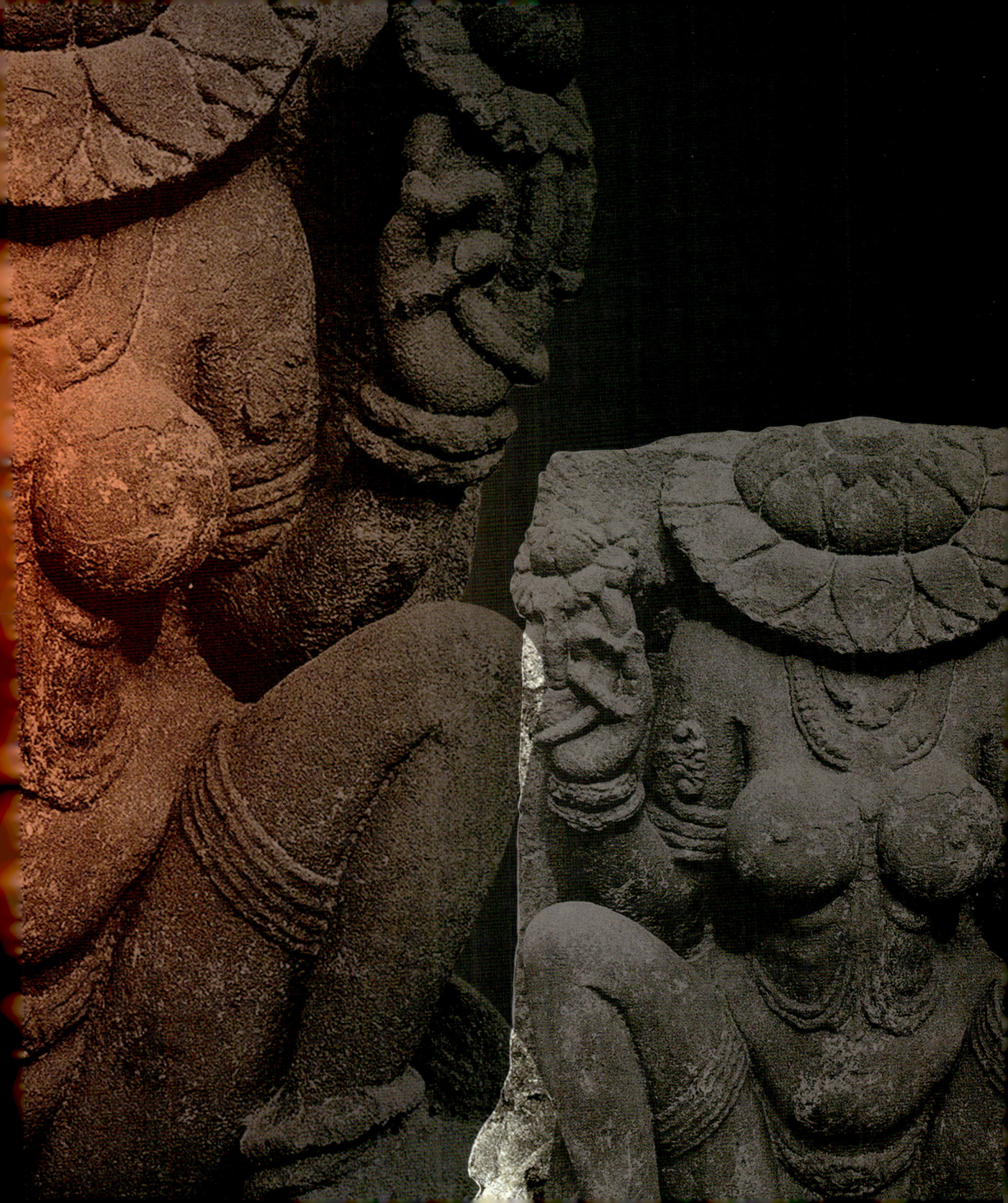

Bibliography

Anon. [Robert Withers?] *A Description of the Grand Signor's Seraglio, or Turkish Emperor's Court*, London, Jo. Martin and Jo. Ridley, 1650.

Artola, George, 'The Transvestite in Sanskrit Story and Drama,' Annals of Oriental Research, 1975.

Ashcroft-Nowicki, Dolores, 'Sex in Ancient Culture': extract from the *Tree of Ecstasy*: *An advanced manual of sexual magic*, Samuel Wieser, York Beach, ME, 1999.

Boswell, J., *Christianity, Social Tolerance and Homosexuality*; University of Chicago Press, Chicago, 1980.

Buchanan, Reverend Robert J., *Homosexuality in History*, Durham, 2000.

Bullough, V.L., *Sexual Variance in Society and History*, University of Chicago Press, Chicago, 1976.

Bullough, V.L. and Bonnie Bullough. *Cross Dressing, Sex, and Gender*, Philadelphia, University of Pennsylvania Press, 1993.

Burkert, W., *Structure and History in Greek Mythology and Ritual*, Berkeley-London, 1979.

Cabezn, Ignacio (ed.), *Buddhism, Sexuality, and Gender*, New York, State University of New York Press.

Chatterjee, Indrani, 'Alienation, Intimacy, and Gender: Problems for a History of Love in South Asia,' in Ruth Vanita (ed.) *Queering India: Same-Sex Love and Eroticism in Indian Culture and Society*, Routledge, New York and London, 2001.

Chaturvedi, Badrinath, *Kama Sutra*, Roli Books, New Delhi, 1999.

Chinese Mythologies, Encyplopedia of glbtq.com

De Silva, A.L., *Homosexuality and Theravada Buddhism*.

Douglas, Nik and Penny Slinger, *Sexual Secrets*, Inner Traditions, US.

Faure, Bernard, *The Red Thread: Buddhist Approaches to Sexuality*. Princeton, NJ, Princeton University Press, 1998.

Goswami, Kanika, *Homosexuality and Our Forefathers*, Buzzle.com, March 2004.

Greek Love J. Z. Eglinton (trans.) Ganymede Books, New York, Oliver Layton Press.

'Greek Mythology: The Legend of Hercules and Zeus, Plutarch and Alexander.' The Androphile Project.

Hall, Kira, 'Hijra/Hijran: Language and Gender Identity.' Unpublished doctoral dissertation, Linguistics, University of California, Berkeley. Ann Arbor, Mich.: UMI, 1995.

Herdt, Gilbert (ed.), *Third Sex, Third Gender: Beyond Sexual Dimorphism in Culture and History*, New York, Zone Books, 1994.

Ijiri Chusuke, 1482, 'The Essence of Jakudo' in *The Love of the Samurai, A Thousand Years of Japanese Homosexuality* by Tsuneo Watanabe and Jun'ichi Iwata, London, The Gay Men's Press, 1989

Jackson, Peter A., 'Essay on Non-normative Sex/Gender Categories in Theravada Buddhist Scriptures,' *Australian Humanities Review*, April 1996.

Jaffrey, Zia, *The Invisibles: The Eunuchs of India*, New York, Vintage Books, 1996.

Joseph, Sherry, 'The Law and Homosexuality in India.' Paper at CEHAT International Conference for preventing Violence, SNDT Mumbai, 1998.

Kautilya, *Arthashastra*, L.N. Rangarajan (trans.), London, Penguin Books, 1992.

Keay, John, *India: A History*, New York, Grove Press, 2000.

Kinsey, Dr Alfred C., *Sexual Behaviour in the Human Male, 1948*. Reprint Indiana University Press, 1998.

Leonard, G., *Education and Ecstasy*, NY, Dell Publishing Co, 1968.

Mahabharata (*Virata Parva*), Kisari Mohan Ganguli, (trans.), 1896.

Manmata Samhita, Sandhya Mulchandani (trans.), 2004.

'Monogamy and Safe Sex,' *Tone Magazine*, November 1999.

Morin, Jack, PhD, *Anal Pleasure and Health: A Guide for Men and Women*, Down There Press, 3rd revised ed., 1998.

Mueller, Max, *Nasadiya Suktam Rg Veda*, Published between 1849 and 1873.

Murray, Stephen O, and Will Roscoe, *Islamic Homosexualities: Culture, History, and Literature*, New York, New York University Press, 1997.

Nanda, Serena, *Neither Man nor Woman: The Hijras of India*. Belmont, CA, Wadsworth, 1990.

Newitz, Annalee, 'Mapping Sexual Geographies.' Essay in Bad Subjects Issue 17 November 1994.

Norman, Stuart, *A New Spirituality for Gays*, 1997.

Pattanaik, Devdutt, *The Man Who Was a Woman and Other Queer Tales from Hindu Lore*, New York, Harrington Park Press, 2002.

Penrose, Walter, 'Hidden in History: Female Homoeroticism and Women of a "Third Nature",' in the *South Asian Past*, Journal of the History of Sexuality 10 : 1 2001.

Plato, *Symposium*, Christopher Gill, Penguin Books, New edition, October 1999.

Rawlinson, H.G., *India: A Short Cultural History*, London, Cresset Press, 1954.

Saletore, Rajaram Narayan, *Sex Life under Indian Rulers*, Delhi, Hind Pocket Books, 1974. Also *Sex in Indian Harem Life*, New Delhi, Orient Paperbacks, 1978.

Sinha, Indra, *Love Teachings of the Kama Sutra*, With Extracts from *Koka Shastra, Ananga Ranga* and Other Famous Indian Works on Love, Indra Sinha, Marlowe and Co., November, 1999.

Swami Prabhupada, *Shrimad Bhagvatam,* (trans.).

Sweet, Michael J., 'Eunuchs, Lesbians and Other Mythical Beasts: Queering and Dequeering the Kama Sutra.'

Sweet, Michael J. and Leonard Zwilling, 'The First Medicalization: The Taxonomy and Etiology of Queerness in Classical Indian Medicine,' *Journal of the History of Sexuality,* April 1993, 3 : 590-607.

———— 'Like a City Ablaze: The Third Sex and the Creation of Sexuality in Jain Religious Literature', Journal of the History of Sexuality, 6 (3): 359-84.

Tantra :The Secret Power of Sex, Kale, Arvind and Shanta, Jaico Publishers, Bombay, 1976.

Thadani, Giti., *Sakhiyani: Lesbian Desire in Ancient and Modern India,* Sexual Politics series, Cassell, London 1996.

The Androphile Project: The World History of Male Love, 2004. www.androphile.org.

The Laws of Manu, Wendy Doniger with Brian K. Smith (trans.), London, Penguin Books, 1991.

The Complete Kama Sutra: The First Unabridged Modern Translation of the Classic Indian Text by Vatsyayana, including the *Jayamangala* commentary by Yashodhara and extracts from the Hindi commentary by Devadatta Shastra. Alain Danielou (trans.), Rochester, Vt.: Park Street Press. 1994.

Vanita, Ruth, (ed.), *Queering India: Same-Sex Love and Eroticism in Indian Culture and Society,* New York, Routledge, 2002.

Vatsyayana, *Kama Sutra of Vatsyayana*: *The Classic Hindu Treatise on Love and Social Conduct.* Translated by Sir Richard S. Burton, Reprint of the 19th century translation, New York, E.P. Dutton, 1963.

Wilber, K., *Up From Eden: A Transpersonal View of Human Evolution*; Shambhala, Boulder, CO, 1982.

Wilhelm, Amara Dasa, *The Third Gender,* published in the Gay and Lesbian Vaishnava Association Inc., Reproduced with permission.

Willis, Roy (ed.), *World Mythology,* New York, Henry Holt Books, Ref BL 311 1993.

Zwilling, Leonard. 'Homosexuality As Seen in Buddhist Texts.' In *Buddhism, Sexuality, and Gender,* edited by Jose Ignacio Cabezon, Albany, State University of New York Press, 1992.

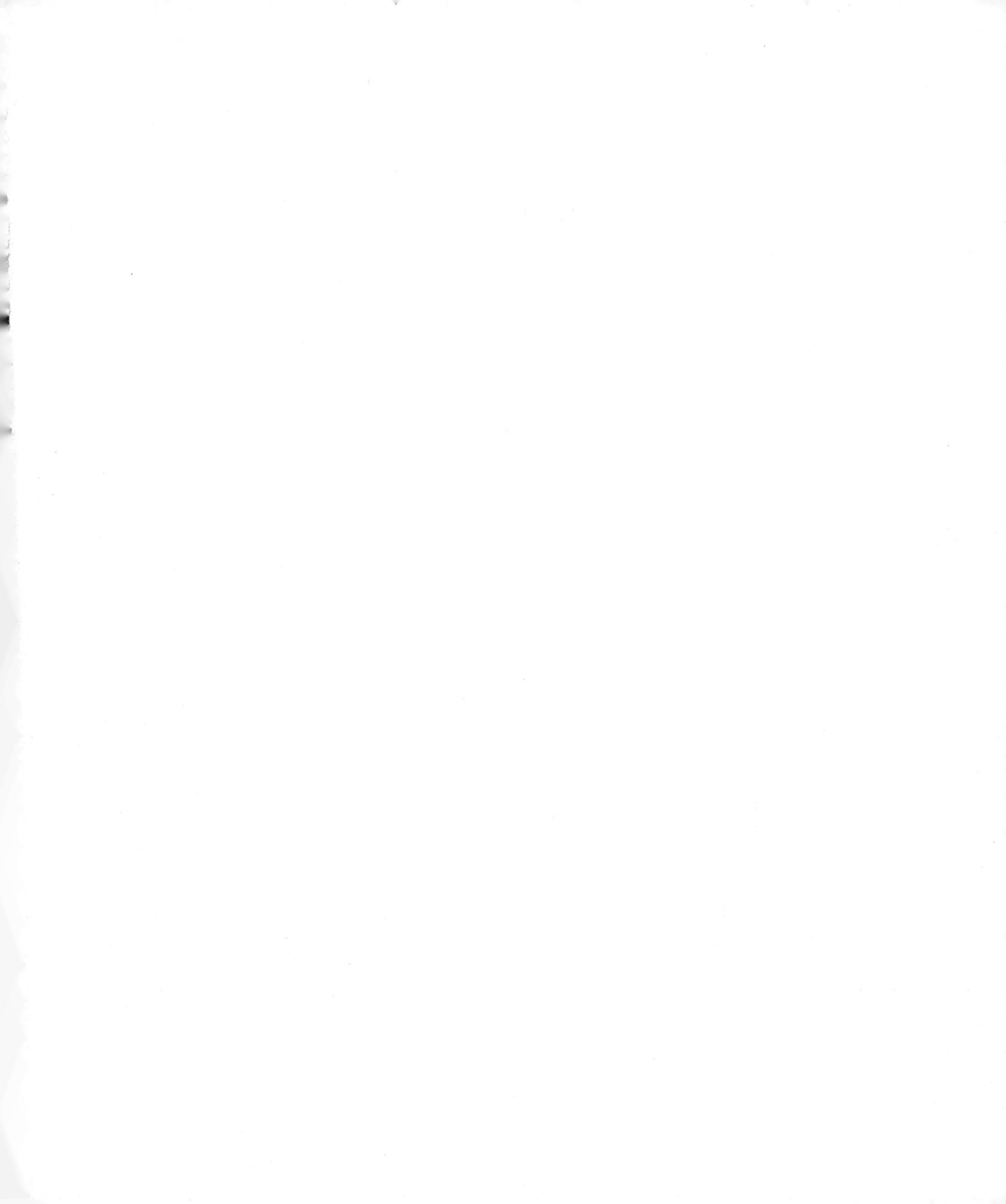